NO MORE
HEART DISEASE

NO MORE
HEART DISEASE

How Nitric Oxide Can Prevent—Even
Reverse—Heart Disease and Stroke

DR. LOUIS J. IGNARRO

St. Martin's Press ≈ New York

www.stmartins.com

Library of Congress Cataloging-in-Publication Data

Ignarro, Louis J.
    No more heart disease : how nitric oxide can prevent—even reverse—heart disease and stroke / by Louis J. Ignarro. —1st U.S. ed.
        p. cm.
    ISBN 0-312-33581-4
    EAN 978-0312-33581-6
    1. Cardiovascular system—Diseases—Popular works. 2. Cardiovascular system—Diseases—Prevention. 3. Nitric oxide—Physiological effect. 4. Dietary supplements. I. Title.

RC672.I135 2005
616.1'05—dc22

                                                    2004051304

10 9 8 7 6 5 4 3 2

This book is dedicated to my wife, Dr. Sharon Ignarro, and my mother, Frances Ignarro. Sharon has been my strongest supporter through all the ups and downs of this wild ride that my discovery, nitric oxide, and the Nobel Prize have taken me on. In addition to being a loving wife, Sharon is also my coach and taskmaster, not to mention a great physician. Without her discipline, I would never have made it to the finish line of the 2004 Los Angeles Marathon at age sixty-two—my first!

My mother, Frances, has been there for every step of my journey to the pinnacle of scientific research. It was Mom's patience and understanding in the early days, when my chemistry experiments were blowing up furniture in our family home, that allowed my scientific curiosity to make it out of the basement and into the research laboratory.

Finally, I especially want to dedicate *NO More Heart Disease* to the sixty million Americans, and millions more around the globe, who suffer from cardiovascular disease. The nitric oxide therapy described in this book can play a significant role in their quest to find cardiovascular wellness.

Because it is important for me to continue my quest for knowledge on the benefits of nitric oxide, I would greatly appreciate it if, after trying my regimen, you could drop me a note with your comments on the benefits of **Say Yes to NO**. You can e-mail me at SayYestoNO@NOMoreHeartDisease.com. Thank you, and enjoy the book.

AUTHOR'S NOTE

The nutrients I recommend in *NO More Heart Disease,* including L-arginine, L-citrulline, and a host of heart-healthy foods, are naturally occurring and generally non-toxic at even very high levels.

Indeed, one of the most attractive properties of nitric oxide and its ability to enhance cardiovascular health is that it does not produce the undesirable side effects that are prevalent with pharmaceuticals. This stands to reason, because nitric oxide is produced in your own bloodstream—by natural nutrients that are found in abundance in the foods all around you.

Nevertheless, you should consult your physician, who is familiar with your personal medical history, before beginning my recommended health regimen—or any other health program, for that matter.

CONTENTS

ACKNOWLEDGMENTS

I was inspired to write this book after I realized that my own basic research and that of my colleagues unraveled new and easy ways to improve and maintain cardiovascular health and overall fitness. Our research on nitric oxide (NO) revealed sufficient knowledge to put every single human being in a position to prevent and to reverse cardiovascular disease. That is, every person now has a choice, a clear choice. When I realized all of this, I tried to think of ways to communicate my beliefs to the millions of people around the world who suffer, many of them unnecessarily, from cardiovascular disease. Certainly, winning the Nobel Prize in Medicine gave me a louder voice to express my views, but primarily to other scientists. What I desperately needed was a way to communicate with everyone. Clearly the answer was to write a book that ordinary people could read and understand. I hope that this book will motivate and help you to attain a level of cardiovascular wellness that will significantly impact your life.

I am sincerely grateful to the many people who contributed to this book. First and foremost, I want to thank Richard Trubo, an accomplished author, who took what I told him and put it into words—very nice and precise words. Without him there would be no book. My thanks go also to Dr. Paul Kirkitelos and Carolyn Fireside, who spent countless hours revising and editing the manuscript so that it could become a book. A book is not complete unless and until the manuscript is proofread and corrected for spelling, grammar, and structure. For this, I express my appreciation and thanks to Arlene Lising Navarro, Laura Brito-McGaha, and Jay Brubaker. Arlene Lising Navarro, my own assistant, made life much easier for me by organizing and handling the dozens of telephone calls, e-mails, and fax transmittals that were necessary to accomplish the task. Also invaluable in this regard was Gina Scarpa at St. Martin's Press. In addition, I would like to thank Michael Dunn for his attention to detail and very thorough follow-up on all matters of importance.

Special thanks go to my business partner, Dave Brubaker. Dave's entrepreneurial spirit and business acumen enabled me not only to tell my story of nitric oxide and cardiovascular health, but also to develop, patent, and bring to market my L-arginine + L-citrulline + antioxidant formula to promote cardiovascular wellness. Thanks to him, thousands of people have already embarked on my simple program to live longer and more productive lives.

My appreciation also goes out to David Vigliano, who believed in what I had to say and made it possible for me to interact with the publisher.

And last but not least, I would like to thank Diane Reverand and St. Martin's Press for believing in the concept of **Say Yes to NO** from the very beginning, and sticking with it until completion.

INTRODUCTION

Winning the 1998 Nobel Prize in Medicine, the culmination of my professional life, confirmed that my decades of research had produced a breakthrough that would profoundly and permanently alter medical science. My colleagues, Ferid Murad and Robert Furchgott, and I had discovered "the atom" of cardiovascular health—a tiny molecule called nitric oxide. NO—as it is known by chemists—is produced by the body specifically to help keep arteries and veins free of the plaque that causes stroke and to maintain normal blood pressure by relaxing the arteries, thereby regulating the rate of blood flow and preventing coronaries. Nitric oxide is the body's natural cardiovascular wonder drug.

As valuable as it is to our health, nitric oxide suffers from an identity crisis. If I asked a roomful of readers like you to tell me what nitric oxide is, most would probably tell me that it is the laughing gas you get at the dentist's office. That is nitro*us* oxide. Others would tell me that nitric oxide is the key ingredient in explosives like dynamite. This time they would be confusing nitric oxide with nitric *acid*. Still others would respond that nitric oxide is contained in cigarette smoke, and is the destructive part of car exhaust that causes smog and acid rain. This final group would be right, although they would be describing what were considered the primary attributes of nitric oxide before my research dramatically changed the scientific world's view of NO. *NO More Heart Disease* will help you to catch up on your understanding of NO.

Our findings could help millions and millions of people—even those already afflicted—to safeguard the health of their hearts and vascular system. So many lives could be saved if we could eradicate heart disease in the foreseeable future.

I have written *NO More Heart Disease* to convey this vitally important information to help you to enjoy a long, high-energy life. By following my simple **Say Yes to NO** regimen to boost your body's production of nitric oxide, you will be taking the first steps to making heart attack and stroke into health plagues of the past. I believe that our findings may someday soon diminish the general incidence of cardiovascular disease beyond the most optimistic projections of medical science even a decade ago.

THE **SAY YES TO NO** PLAN—A REAL LIFESAVER!

By embarking on my three-tiered plan for age-proofing your cardiovascular system with enhanced NO production, you can lower your blood pressure and keep your vascular network clean and elastic. You will be nourishing every cell in your body without making extreme lifestyle adjustments—simply by incorporating NO-friendly foods into your daily diet, taking specifically targeted supplements, and maintaining a moderate, nontaxing fitness program tailored to your specific health and wellness needs.

Each part of the program exerts a substantial positive influence on your cardiovascular health, but when they are employed together in the **Say Yes to NO Plan,** the result is very powerful due to a process called synergy. The whole in this case is greater than the sum of its parts—as each element of the plan contributes not only to NO production, but also to the effectiveness of the other parts' ability to increase NO production.

A critical example of the NO-producing synergy contained in the **Say Yes to NO Plan** is my recommendation for the amino acids L-arginine and L-citrulline, combined with four key antioxidants. My research shows that if you take only L-arginine, which is the dominant producer of NO, you will not receive the maximum benefit. I have found that by including the synergistic partner L-citrulline, your ability to boost NO production is greatly enhanced over the effects of L-arginine alone. The same is true of the antioxidants, which synergize L-arginine by protecting the NO from oxidation once it has been produced, thereby ensuring that it can be effectively used by the body.

Any supplement program that does not contain L-citrulline and antioxidants to augment the L-arginine—and most on the market do not—is missing out on a major piece of the potential of NO to improve your cardiovascular health. My **Say Yes to NO Plan** is uniquely effective because of its synergistic combination of L-arginine, L-citrulline, and antioxidants.

It is clear to see that the best results will come from adhering as closely as possible to the details of the **Say Yes to NO Plan**. All in all, the minor lifestyle changes required to boost your NO production and nourish your cells are a small price to pay for the huge payoff of a better chance at a longer, healthier life.

Warning: Don't Be Fooled by Impostors!

Do not let yourself be confused by the growing number of products on the market that simply promise to deliver "nitric oxide." They are by and large scientifically questionable attempts to boost your NO without accurately applying my Nobel Prize–winning discoveries. These products often contain L-arginine, which is indeed the amino acid that is converted by your body into NO. Unfortunately, most of them do not deliver sufficient quantities of L-arginine to catalyze significant NO production. My **Say Yes to NO Plan** prescribes L-arginine in doses (4 to 6 grams a day) that have been rigorously proven in the laboratory to boost NO considerably, thereby producing maximum cardiovascular health benefits. Few products on the market contain this level of L-arginine. My research shows that L-arginine in doses smaller than 4 to 6 grams produces almost zero increase in NO, so it is in essence an "all or nothing" proposition—you must receive the full dose of L-arginine.

Besides insufficient doses of L-arginine, other products completely miss the point of the breakthroughs that you are about to learn in my **Say Yes to NO** program. *It is the synergy between the L-arginine (in a large enough dose), the L-citrulline, and the key antioxidants that creates dramatic increases in your body's nitric oxide production.* Without the proper combination of these nutrients, which so many other programs lack, you will receive little or no benefit from NO therapy.

> Before you purchase any product that is billed as a NO booster, check the nutritional data carefully. If the ingredients do not measure up to the prescription in *NO More Heart Disease,* you are wasting your time and money while missing the chance to improve your cardiovascular health. In that case, just say "NO!," and stick with the facts contained in the pages that follow.

WHO CAN BENEFIT FROM THIS BOOK?

The program described in this book is beneficial for many different types of readers. For those adults who have already suffered cardiovascular damage—typically people over fifty, although damage has unfortunately become more common in young people as well—the program can help you reverse its effects. For those who have not yet suffered significant damage, the book provides a powerful heart disease prevention program, helping you safeguard your body from the effects of aging and other factors in heart disease.

The book is *as much for women as it is for men,* although pregnant and lactating women may have different considerations and should always consult their physicians. Despite many preconceived notions, heart disease is no longer exclusively the province of men. Heart disease claims the lives of some 8.6 million women every year and is now the number-one killer of women, outpacing even cancer. Although women have a higher mortality rate from heart disease, men are still the prime target, as evidenced by their higher risk of contracting the disease, particularly at younger ages. This book crosses gender lines, offering a vital prescription for both men and women through my **Say Yes to NO** program.

The science in *NO More Heart Disease* is as direct as it can be, because I am the scientist who discovered it. Ever since the Nobel committee saw fit to reward these breakthroughs with the prize, I have been on a nearly ceaseless journey, explaining the information in a way that nonscientists can understand and apply. The presentation in this book is designed to give you the facts in a straightforward manner, avoiding the scientific jargon and other complexities that could obscure the main points.

NO More Heart Disease begins with the story of NO, which is the story of Alfred Nobel, Lou Ignarro, and a century-long process that ended in a major breakthrough in cardiovascular health. After the story of the research, I teach you how your cardiovascular system functions and malfunctions, followed by some of the practical applications of the nitric oxide discovery. Next I explain the role of NO in each of the four essential bodily processes—vascular tone, coagulation, inflammation, and oxidation.

Starting in Chapter 5, the book dives into my *Say Yes to NO* age-proofing regimen, introducing and briefly explaining the supplement package, the dietary recommendations, and the fitness guidelines. I then take you through each of the three branches of the program, backing every supplemental, nutritional, and fitness suggestion with solid science. The tour concludes with Dr. Ignarro's **Say Yes to NO** Regimen in a Nutshell, designed as a quick reference as you apply the program in your own life.

Threaded through *NO More Heart Disease* are testimonials from men and women all over America, who have seen their well-being improve enormously with NO therapy. I have also included case histories and sidebars of salient information, including academic studies of NO. I conclude with final thoughts, in which I tell you about the very latest in NO research as well as the potentially dramatic future breakthroughs that will help us all to enjoy better cardiovascular health.

THE NO BENEFITS THAT AWAIT YOU

My **Say Yes to NO** program has the potential to restore the normal production and activity of nitric oxide in your body, and in turn, improve your cardiovascular health. Following my plan will:

- lower your blood pressure
- improve your circulation
- delay the onset or progression of atherosclerosis
- reduce your likelihood of (and possibly prevent) having a heart attack or a stroke

These are not unfounded, unsubstantiated claims. Grounded in science, these claims are supported by studies in my own lab at the UCLA School of Medicine and by many other research scientists around the world.

No matter what your age or physical condition, you can put your body's NO to work effectively by adopting my recommendations.

When you **Say Yes to NO,** you do your heart and body good.

NO MORE
HEART DISEASE

1

EUREKA!
MY PERSONAL JOURNEY
FROM A. NOBEL TO THE NOBEL

PRESS RELEASE:

The 1998 Nobel Prize in Physiology or Medicine

NOBELFÖRSAMLINGEN KAROLINSKA INSTITUTET
THE NOBEL ASSEMBLY AT KAROLINSKA INSTITUTET

October 12, 1998

The Nobel Assembly at Karolinska Institutet has today decided to award the Nobel Prize in Physiology or Medicine for 1998 to Robert F. Furchgott, Louis J. Ignarro, and Ferid Murad for their discoveries concerning "nitric oxide as a signalling molecule in the cardiovascular system."

When I shared the 1998 Nobel Prize in Medicine with Robert F. Furchgott and Ferid Murad, I was overjoyed that the honor would bring NO to the forefront of worldwide scientific awareness. Being awarded the Nobel Prize was also the culmination of my personal journey from a scientifically curious childhood in New York to the world's most prestigious science award—a journey guided every step of the way by that titan of science and industry, Alfred Nobel. One reason my Nobel Prize was so noteworthy is that there exists a genuine scientific connection between my nitric oxide discoveries and Nobel's life and work involving the same molecule. In a very direct way, Nobel planted the seed in my mind that grew into my obsession with studying the little-known substance.

THE LIFE AND WORK OF ALFRED NOBEL

A brilliant nineteenth-century Swedish chemist and inventor as well as a skillful industrialist, Alfred Nobel held 355 patents, one of which was for dynamite, a powdery mixture using nitroglycerin as its active ingredient. Nobel built factories in twenty countries, manufacturing and selling large quantities of dynamite to construction and mining companies as well as the military. The availability of dynamite transformed the construction industry, because it could be used to blast through hills and mountains and to clear pathways for roads, bridges, tunnels, and dams.

Nobel knew all too well that liquid nitroglycerin would sometimes explode unexpectedly when subjected to heat or pressure. His own twenty-one-year-old brother, Emil, and four other people were killed in an explosion at one of the family's manufacturing plants. Years earlier, Asciano Sobrero, the Italian chemist who invented nitroglycerin in 1846, suffered severe scarring of his face in a nitroglycerin explosion.

Since Stockholm's city officials banned nitroglycerin research within the city limits, Nobel was forced to conduct his experiments on a barge anchored on a nearby lake. Eventually, he discovered that by using silica, an additive similar to sand, with nitroglycerin, he could employ dynamite safely without the fear of accidental explosions.

Nobel's attentiveness to the details of his business led him to recognize an unusual phenomenon occurring in his factories. Many workers complained of developing severe headaches on Monday mornings when they returned to work after the weekend—only to have the headaches subside over the following weekend. The headaches were traced to the factory's use of nitroglycerin, a volatile substance whose fumes dilate blood vessels, increasing blood flow to the brain. Those fumes triggered throbbing headaches, because they caused "vascular instability"—the dilation and/or constriction of the blood vessels to the brain. Nobel himself suffered from migraines, which may have been related to his contact with nitroglycerin.

At the same time, some of Nobel's factory employees reported that their angina pain subsided on workdays when they were in close proximity to nitroglycerin, only to worsen when they were away from the factory. Again, it was almost certainly the nitroglycerin fumes that were responsible for their chest-pain relief.

Coincidentally, physicians in the late nineteenth century had found that small doses of nitroglycerin were useful in the management of chest discomfort, although no one knew exactly how it worked. When Nobel himself developed heart disease and angina pain in the 1890s—so severe that it often left him bedridden—he stubbornly disregarded his doctor's orders to take nitroglycerin, refusing to believe that such a powerful explosive could have any medical value. In a letter to a friend, written several months before his death from heart disease in 1896, Nobel wrote: "My heart trouble will keep me here in Paris for another few days at least. . . . Isn't it the irony of fate that I have been prescribed nitroglycerin to be taken internally! They call it Trinitrin, so as not to scare the chemist and the public."

If Nobel had had more faith in nitroglycerin as a vasodilator, his life may well have been prolonged. Before he died, he laid the groundwork for the awarding of the Nobel Prizes, hoping history would remember him as more than the man who invented dynamite, one of the most destructive substances in the world of his time.

FROM BROOKLYN TO STOCKHOLM

It seems unlikely that the story of Nobel's life could be so intimately connected to mine. We certainly came from vastly different beginnings and different times. Were it not for Nobel's genius and the work that it produced, my life and work would have taken an entirely different course. As it turned out, fate seemed to bring Nobel and me together in the name of science.

I am the son of Italian immigrant parents who came to the United States in the 1920s—poor in terms of money and education, but rich in hope. They met and married in Brooklyn in the 1930s, where I was born on May 31, 1941. My brother, Angelo, and I were raised in a beautiful seaside community on the South Shore of Long Island called Long Beach. My father supported the family as a carpenter.

Papa would occasionally take me to work with him so I could watch him do his carpentry, but when I was ten, he stopped inviting me along. I think he was afraid that I might choose to become a laborer like him rather than go to college. He must have regarded my relentless demand for a chemistry set when I was eight as a sign that I was headed toward a less physically demanding profession. That chemistry set became my prized possession as I improvised my way through one experiment after another.

As I progressed to larger chemistry sets and more challenging experiments, I decided that what I really wanted to do was build a small firecrackerlike bomb. Before long, my ambition led me to the public library, where I read everything on the shelves about explosives and fuel and took pages and pages of handwritten notes about what I was reading. I often encountered the name and work of Alfred Nobel, and I was fascinated both by his work in explosives and by the connection between nitroglycerin and angina relief.

As I read about Nobel's career, I was even more inspired to create something explosive. I experimented for months. I not only used chemicals from my chemistry sets, but also persuaded some older boys in the neighborhood to obtain other chemicals for me from the local pharmacy. My attempt at making a firecracker inadvertently turned into much more—a pipe bomb that destroyed a piece of furniture in my house and caused my mother great distress.

Before long I turned from bomb-making to rocket science. I launched a homemade rocket in the backyard that, on its descent, landed on our roof and shattered tiles as it crash-landed. My father was as impressed with my progress as he was angry about the roof. His lenient attitude toward my interest in science allowed me to continue to pursue this passion, ultimately pointing me in the direction that my life would take.

I attended Columbia University and took every chemistry course I could find, although a class in pharmacology really piqued my interest. In graduate school at the University of Minnesota I studied pharmacology with a minor in cardiovascular physiology—another debt I owe to my reading on Nobel. With my Ph.D. in hand, I set out to identify and solve some of the mysteries of medicine and pharmacology.

When I began my career as a pharmacologist, my childhood fascination with the link between nitroglycerin and relief of angina came to the fore. Before long, my research was beginning to move slowly but surely toward NO. Having studied a molecule called cyclic guanosine monophosphate (GMP), which appeared to be another important vascular smooth muscle relaxant, I became intrigued by the research of Houston pharmacologist Ferid Murad. At the time, Murad was conducting some of the earliest studies of nitric oxide. Until then, only chemists seemed interested in NO as a reactive chemical. He and his colleagues wrote a paper that captured my attention, because it showed that NO could not only activate the enzyme that produces cyclic GMP, but could also increase the concentration of cyclic GMP in human tissues by a hundred times. Meanwhile in New York, pharmacologist Robert F. Furchgott was drawing some conclusions that dovetailed with Murad's and mine, but that story will come later.

The question was whether NO could be doing something beneficial in the body. Almost a century later scientists and physicians still shared Alfred Nobel's grave reservations about nitroglycerin and its chemical relatives, finding it inconceivable that NO could play a positive role in the human body. After all, NO was a toxic substance—a component of auto exhaust and cigarette smoke—in short, a major environmental pollutant. How could it heal? I did not yet have all the answers, but I had a hunch, and I intended to continue acting on it.

NO TAKES THE STAGE

Another key question had to be answered. Could compounds like nitroglycerin relieve chest pain by working through a NO mechanism? Even though nitroglycerin had been used for more than a hundred years to dilate the blood vessels of people whose heart muscle was deprived of oxygen, its mechanism of action was still not known. Certainly the drug did not work by causing little explosions in the blood vessels. So what was the mechanism?

Ferid Murad suspected that the "nitro" portion of nitroglycerin might be converted to NO in the smooth muscle walls of blood vessels, and that NO caused the smooth muscle of the vessels to relax. We were not sure this hypothesis could be proven in a laboratory, but I wanted to test it to see if Murad was right. I shifted the pace of my experiments and data-gathering into overdrive. The research was meticulous, and there were no instant breakthroughs. Ultimately the evidence, once thought to be improbable, gradually fell into place and clearly defined the way that nitroglycerin works.

From the start, NO was a challenging molecule to study. We had to purchase the NO gas in tanks and conduct our experiments while wearing masks and hoods to protect us from caustic substances. Since NO is very unstable and is converted to nitrate and nitrite within seconds, we had to dilute it with nitrogen or argon, which preserve and keep it from decomposing in no more than a millisecond. We used gas-tight syringes and injected the NO gas into an "organ bath" resembling human blood and containing blood vessels. At times our experiments began to look like science fiction, and the scientific majority continued to believe they were—until we were able to measure a marked relaxation of the blood vessels' vascular smooth muscles triggered by nitric oxide. It was the first proof of just how important NO would turn out to be, and it became the springboard for the twenty-four years of studies that ensued.

My studies showed that when an angina patient takes nitroglycerin, it triggers an irreversible domino effect within the body. As the nitroglycerin enters the blood vessels, it is converted inside the vascular tissue into a short-lived gas called nitric oxide. NO stimulates the formation of cyclic GMP, which acts as a messenger carrying instructions for the blood vessels to relax and widen. The result is a greater flow of blood and oxygen to the heart, a decrease in chest pains, and a decline in blood pressure readings.

THE MESSENGER SERVICE WITHIN US

The importance of NO had become clear, but as my research progressed, new questions continued to arise. For example, why did our bodies have the built-in mechanism or the receptors to respond to an outside chemical like nitroglycerin? How did the body know how to react? One theory was that humans might produce our own naturally occurring NO—in a sense, our own form of nitroglycerin—that functions as a signaling molecule specifically to control blood pressure. I have always believed that if the body is able to respond to an outside chemical, that chemical may already exist in the body. If that was true, and if our bodies could be stimulated to produce all the NO we need, would there even be a need for treatments like nitroglycerin?

Although this hypothesis made sense to me, I felt like a lone voice among my scientist colleagues. Most simply never considered the possibility that NO could be a naturally occurring molecule, which was actually beneficial to cardiovascular health rather than just being nontoxic at the proper level. I turned my attention to either confirming or refuting the theory that the body itself—in particular, our own blood vessels—makes nitric oxide.

Before long, the results proved very exciting. We conducted the first studies to confirm that nitroglycerin could be converted in the test tube—and in the body—to NO, and that we have our own form of nitroglycerin stored as NO in the body to regulate blood pressure and blood clotting. At extraordinarily high concentrations, NO is toxic. These levels, however, cannot be reached through the body's internal mechanisms for producing NO from either food and supplement intake or from exercise. At relatively low levels within the body—the kind that *can* be attained through foods, supplements, and exercise—NO can dramatically influence our health in positive ways.

A PARALLEL TRACK

I mentioned another fascinating NO breakthrough earlier, which is a critical piece of the NO puzzle, this one involving my co-laureate Robert Furchgott.

Although nitric oxide became the focus of my own research in 1978, the major breakthrough in our understanding of its healing properties did not come until 1986. Until then, I had conducted studies evaluating the properties of NO in an attempt to solve many unanswered questions, including why the body has its own internal mechanism for responding to this gas. At the same time, a parallel track of research had been launched by Dr. Robert Furchgott at the State University of New York in Brooklyn, although he did not focus specifically on NO.

In 1980, Furchgott and his colleagues discovered the existence of a signaling or messenger molecule manufactured within the endothelial cells lining the blood vessels causing them to relax. Since the endothelium had not previously been thought to play a major role in vascular dilation, Furchgott's finding was particularly intriguing to researchers like me. The molecule remained unidentified for years. Like NO, it was a difficult substance to study, because it was remarkably short-lived.

Because it existed for less than a second, no one was able to pin down and isolate its chemical structure.

Furchgott, feeling he had to assign a name to the enigmatic substance, chose to label it endothelium-derived relaxing factor, or EDRF. We agreed that, once we decoded its molecular structure, EDRF could help us design experiments to determine the causes of cardiovascular disease—and perhaps develop new methods to prevent, even reverse it.

By 1986, I began to entertain the possibility that EDRF might actually be nitric oxide. Until that time, there was no reason to suspect that EDRF and NO were the same substance. I designed a series of experiments comparing the properties of EDRF and NO. I reviewed my lab notebooks repeatedly. I dissected my data again and again. I set aside everything else I was doing in the lab and worked around the clock on the NO/EDRF resemblance.

Every experiment led me to the same conclusion: NO was, in fact, the elusive compound EDRF, which shared all its properties with NO. They both dilated the blood vessels, were very unstable, and had extremely brief life spans. I had no doubts about the clinical significance of NO and EDRF being the same substance. Based on what we knew about EDRF, nitric oxide's role in the body became much clearer: It was definitely a signaling molecule, which performed crucial cardiovascular functions in the body.

Within weeks, I presented my NO/EDRF data at a conference of prominent vascular researchers at the Mayo Clinic, and the reception was, well, underwhelming. The audience was clearly skeptical. I was beginning to feel I was the only person in the auditorium who believed my results. After I had finished, someone jokingly suggested perhaps I had inhaled a little too much NO before I walked up to the podium. I could not understand their doubts, because the data were irrefutable.

SCIENCE SEES THE LIGHT

It was never a simple path to the acceptance of our nitric oxide discoveries. When we had first attempted to publish our research showing that nitroglycerin works through the actions of NO, our work was rejected by more than one major scientific journal. Fortunately, many scientists did recognize the importance of the work. As the pace of my own NO research intensified, our studies eventually were published.

At that point, the skeptics were still critical, but the nature of their objection had changed. They claimed that even though NO had turned out to be the active ingredient in nitroglycerin, it probably would not prove important in other areas. When my ongoing studies confirmed that NO could also interfere with the blood clotting that can trigger heart attacks and strokes and could reduce blood pressure, even the naysayers finally had to acknowledge that NO appeared to have enormous health implications.

By 1986, our studies repeatedly showed that the body could make its own NO. My hypothesis proved true—the endothelial cells of blood vessels can produce NO for the purposes of controlling blood pressure. And now that my findings were coalescing with Furchgott's, proving that the endothelium-derived relaxing factor was really NO, the scientific community began to believe that my conclusions were valid.

By 1990, our experiments indicated that NO is also the chemical messenger responsible for penile erections. Nerves in the erectile tissues release NO, dilating the blood vessels and initiating erections. The discovery soon led to the development and marketing by Pfizer of the drug Viagra, which in 2003 had annual global sales of $1.8 billion. The success of this drug led some of my friends to call me "The Father of Viagra." (I have also been referred to as "Dr. NO.")

Our discoveries about blood pressure, blood clotting, and erectile dysfunction were only the start. Low levels of NO are associated with many of the most common diseases of mankind—from infections to malignancies to diabetic complications. We found that NO influences the functioning and well-being of the entire body.

The Nobel Committee Recognizes the Remarkable Power of Nitric Oxide

The Nobel Committee's press release announcing the 1998 award in medicine for the breakthrough research on NO outlined the many functions carried out by the "Miracle Molecule" NO. The following is an excerpt from the press release:

Heart: In atherosclerosis, the endothelium has a reduced capacity to produce NO. However, NO can be furnished by treatment with nitroglycerin. Large efforts in drug discovery are currently aimed at generating more powerful and selective cardiac drugs based on the new knowledge of NO as a signal molecule.

Lungs: Intensive care patients can be treated by inhalation of NO gas. This has provided good results and even saved lives. For instance, NO gas has been used to reduce dangerously high blood pressure in the lungs of infants. But the dosage is critical since the gas can be toxic at high concentrations.

<u>Cancer:</u> White blood cells use NO not only to kill infectious agents such as bacteria, fungi, and parasites, but also to defend the host against tumors. Scientists are currently testing whether NO can be used to stop the growth of tumors since this gas can induce programmed cell death, apoptosis.

<u>Impotence:</u> NO can initiate erection of the penis by dilating the blood vessels to the erectile bodies. This knowledge has already led to the development of new drugs against impotence.

<u>Diagnostic Analyses:</u> Inflammatory diseases can be revealed by analyzing the production of NO from, e.g., the lungs and intestines. This is used for diagnosing asthma, colitis, and other diseases.

<u>Other Functions:</u> NO is important for the olfactory sense and our capacity to recognize different scents. It may even be important for our memory.

—Nobel Assembly at Karolinska Institutet, announcement of 1998 Nobel Prize in Medicine. October 12, 1998.

IS THIS SOMEBODY'S IDEA OF A JOKE?

In August 1998, I was en route from the south of France to a speaking engagement at the University of Naples, Italy. As I waited in line to board a connecting flight at the Nice airport, I was paged. The airline employee handed me a mobile phone and told me I had a call from the United States, cautioning me to make it brief, because I had to board in less than a minute.

I hit the talk button and heard a familiar voice say "Lou, this is Robin." Robin Farias-Eisner, a surgical oncologist at UCLA, is a close friend, but I was baffled. Why would he be calling me at three-thirty in the morning L.A. time, and how had he tracked me down? My first thought was that something had happened to my family, my second that Los Angeles had suffered a major earthquake. But Robin didn't seem the least bit upset.

After a few seconds of small talk, he paused, then practically shouted, "Lou, I have something to tell you. You've just been awarded the Nobel Prize in Medicine!"

"What?" Before he had a chance to tell me more, we were disconnected, and the gate agent was ordering me to board the plane immediately.

During the short flight to Naples, my mind raced, trying to process what I had just heard. I knew that the Nobel Prizes were announced each October, and this was October 12. I did not think that Robin would have tracked me down in Nice just to play a practical joke. As I was waiting my turn to disembark after the plane landed in Naples, I was surprised to see my friend Giuseppe Cirino, a professor of pharmacology who had invited me to Naples, standing on the tarmac at the foot the stairs. Beside him was a crowd of photographers, all aiming their cameras at the plane. When I started down the steps, I was greeted by a torrent of flashing cameras, and I wondered who was behind me.

As soon as I reached Giuseppe, he asked, "Lou, have you heard the news?"

"What news?" Could it actually be possible? Could what Robin had said be true?

Giuseppe handed me a press release issued by the Karolinska Institutet, the medical center at which the Nobel Prize winners are selected. Although the document was written in Swedish, I saw the five-letter word "NOBEL"—and as I scanned the page, I spotted my name. I was overcome. Knocked cold by a one-two punch of disbelief and astonishment, I fell to my knees on the hard concrete of the tarmac. Giuseppe and several airline employees had to help me get inside the terminal.

When I finally composed myself, it occurred to me that I had learned about winning the Nobel Prize in Naples, the birthplace of my late father, who had always encouraged me to develop my scientific curiosity. That is when the tears came.

On a frigid, snow-driven December evening in 1998, the one hundred and second anniversary of Alfred Nobel's death, I found myself in the Stockholm Concert Hall, sharing the stage with King Carl XVI Gustaf, wearing tails and rows of decorations, Queen Silvia nearby in a peach-colored gown, and my two co-laureates. Since each Nobel laureate is allowed to invite fifteen to twenty guests, I had asked many of the scientists and researchers who had worked in my lab over the years to join me. When my turn came, I rose from an oversized red chair to receive the prize, a gold medallion, and a certificate, bowing to the king as trumpets played.

Although there were many extraordinary moments during my ten days in Stockholm, the significance of the Nobel Prize really struck me on my last day there. I was asked to sign my name to a book that contained the signatures of all the Nobel laureates in every field, dating back to 1901. Before adding my own signature on the first empty page in the book, I spent a few minutes slowly turning the pages. As I recognized one famous name after another—a virtual who's who in the fields of medicine, physics, chemistry, and literature—I felt humbled.

There was Ivan Pavlov, who won the award in 1904 . . . Rudyard Kipling in 1907 . . . Madame Curie in 1903 and 1911 . . . Albert Einstein in 1921 . . . George Bernard Shaw in

1926 . . . Sinclair Lewis in 1930 . . . Sir Alexander Fleming in 1945 . . . William Faulkner in 1950 . . . Sir Winston Churchill in 1953 . . . Ernest Hemingway in 1954 . . . Linus Pauling in 1954 and 1962 . . . John Steinbeck in 1962. As my gaze moved down one page, then the next, I asked myself, "Do I really belong in the company of these great men and women?" I was honored that the Nobel Committee believed that I did.

Since few people believed in my ideas at the outset, I often had difficulty funding my initial NO research in the late seventies and early eighties. Representatives of the National Institutes of Health and other funding organizations informed me that, though my research may have been interesting biochemically, they could not understand where I was taking it. With funds limited, they were hesitant to give me money if the medical significance of my work was not clear.

At that time there were very few research papers being published about NO—only about forty per year—and many of those came from my own lab. As our studies got more and more attention, they jump-started a tidal wave of NO research around the world. Some of it was basic laboratory research; other investigators, including me, were exploring the role of NO in protecting the cardiovascular system against hypertension, heart disease, stroke, and atherosclerosis, as well as helping sufferers of gastrointestinal ulcers, sexual dysfunction, and the vascular complications of diabetes.

For years, large and small discoveries about NO have been made on almost a weekly basis. By 2001, as a result of the Nobel Prize, the yearly number of papers published about NO had soared to more than 7,500. That figure continues to climb, with a growing number of scientists entering a field that was virtually neglected just a few years ago. There is even a new scientific journal devoted exclusively to NO. It's called *Nitric Oxide,* and I am proud to say I was its first editor.

Yes, it was exciting to win the Nobel Prize and see the field of NO research explode. Even more exhilarating is the certainty that our research has been used to improve the health of so many men and women. I think Alfred Nobel would be pleased, even impressed, that nitroglycerin, the same substance he feared was solely an agent of destruction, should have proved the key to discoveries that would help men and women around the globe lead healthier and longer lives.

2

YOUR CARDIOVASCULAR SYSTEM: AN OWNER'S MANUAL

In order for you to understand how NO protects your cardiovascular system, you must first gain a basic knowledge of how that system works—and what happens when it breaks down. If you are like most people, you will not give much thought to your cardiovascular system until something goes wrong with it. The endurance, stamina, and complexity of the system are staggering. Every part of your body needs oxygen and nutrients to stay alive, and your cardiovascular system delivers them in an elegant, efficient manner twenty-four hours a day.

Since nitric oxide is crucial to the well-being of your cardiovascular system, it is important for you to know why the nourishment of the cells of your heart and blood vessels with NO is an absolute health necessity.

THE CENTER OF THE ACTION

Your cardiovascular system is composed of the heart and blood vessels, with your heart at the center of the action. The heart is a four-chambered muscular pump, a little larger than a man's fist, and like the workaholic that it is, it never takes a breather.

For seventy, eighty or more years, your heart beats slightly more than once each second, contracting and then propelling about three ounces per beat of freshly oxygenated blood into your aorta, the large blood vessel attached to your heart muscle. The blood then winds its way into your body's vascular system, including the coronary arteries, which embrace the heart and send the blood farther on in its travels.

In addition to the arteries, which carry oxygen-rich blood away from the heart, your network of blood vessels includes the veins and the capillaries. The veins carry oxygen-depleted blood back to the heart for replenishment, and the capillaries connect to the arteries and veins. The circulating blood can be likened to a river that flows through an intricate system of arteries and veins so immense that, if you were to lay them end-to-end, they would extend for 100,000 miles. Think of it. Your vascular network is more than twice as large as the circumference of the earth, yet your blood makes a complete voyage through the body about once a minute.

Clearly the cardiovascular system plays a powerful regulatory role in every major bodily function and organ—more specifically, every cell in the body. If the system is compromised, if vessels become constricted and hardening plaque builds up in them, you become a prime candidate for heart attack and stroke, often without noticeable symptoms.

As the heart beats, dependably and heroically about 100,000 times a day, it pumps nearly 2,000 gallons of blood throughout your body every twenty-four hours. Your heart speeds up during exercise, and slows down during rest, yet it always presses on. At its healthiest, your cardiovascular system works with unwavering precision to deliver what the body requires. That is at optimal function. For millions of people, heart health is far from optimal.

The Sobering Stats on Cardiovascular Disease (CVD)

from The National Institutes of Health and The Centers for Disease Control

- Since 1900, cardiovascular disease has been the number one killer in the United States every year except 1918, the year of the great influenza epidemic.

- Cardiovascular disease claims as many lives each year as the next seven leading causes of death combined.

- There were 65,827,000 physician office visits with the primary diagnosis of cardiovascular disease in 1999.

- Nearly 62 million Americans have at least one type of cardiovascular disease, including high blood pressure, coronary heart disease, angina pectoris (chest pain due to insufficient blood flow through the heart), and stroke.

- Every twenty-nine seconds, an American has what doctors call a "coronary event," such as a heart attack. A death occurs from these events about once every minute.

- Cardiovascular disease claimed 958,775 lives in the United States in 1999—40.1 percent of all deaths.

- Every fifty-three seconds, someone in the United States has a stroke. A death from a stroke takes place every three minutes.

- More people visit their doctor's office for hypertension, or high blood pressure, than for any other reason.

- Cardiovascular disease affects women as well as men. Women actually outnumber men in the prevalence of cases of cardiovascular disease and in related deaths, with about 53 percent of the deaths from cardiovascular disease occurring in women. Although studies repeatedly show that women are much more anxious about developing breast cancer than cardiovascular disease, one of every 2.4 deaths in women is caused by cardiovascular disease, compared to one in thirty from breast cancer.

- In 2001, the economic cost of all cardiovascular disease was approximately $298 billion, including health expenditures and lost productivity. More than $28 billion was spent on cardiovascular drugs.

- In the United States each year, cardiologists perform more than 900,000 angioplasties and surgeons perform more than 121,000 carotid endarterectomies to help prevent stroke.

- Strokes and heart attacks are among the leading causes of long-term chronic disability.

- Up to 90 percent of all cases of impotence are now known to be directly related to "vascular insufficiency."

MOST CARDIOVASCULAR DISEASE DOESN'T HAVE TO HAPPEN

Woody Allen once observed that no one gets out of this world alive. As you can see, too many people are leaving this earth prematurely because of cardiovascular disease. According to the Centers for Disease Control and Prevention, if all types of cardiovascular disease were eradicated, Americans would live an average of nearly seven years longer. Imagine adding seven years to your life expectancy. This, of course, is where NO can help. The best defense is a good offense. If you can elevate your levels of NO—which the program in this book will show you how to do—you can increase your chances of better health and a longer life. With the use of the strategies in this book to boost your NO levels, most cases of cardiovascular disease can be prevented.

PROFILING CARDIOVASCULAR DISEASES

When you hear the words "cardiovascular disease," do you automatically think of heart attacks? Most people do, although as I have already explained, cardiovascular disease covers a much wider scope of serious health problems. Heart attacks are just one type of cardiovascular disease. Fortunately, NO can positively affect virtually all of them.

Here is a little more background on the most common forms of cardiovascular disease:

High Blood Pressure

You have probably had your blood pressure taken many times. When your doctor wraps a cuff around your arm and determines your pressure, he is measuring the force that your blood exerts against the walls of your arteries as it moves through the circulatory system. Your doctor is interested in two important numbers: The *systolic* pressure is the force on your arterial walls as your heart beats or contracts to pump out blood. Your blood pressure is at its highest when it beats. By contrast, the *diastolic* pressure is the pressure on the walls as your heart relaxes between beats and fills with blood.

The Hypertension Epidemic

More people visit their doctor's office for hypertension (high blood pressure) than for any other reason. In fact, a startling 50 million Americans have high blood pressure. Even so, about 32 percent of the people with hypertension are not even aware that they have it, and another 26 percent are taking blood pressure-lowering medications, all of which have side effects, but still do not have their hypertension under control.

Why Pressure Soars To understand high blood pressure, picture a garden hose with a nozzle on its tip. There are two ways to increase the water pressure. Either you can open the faucet and pump more water through the hose, or you can tighten the nozzle and increase the resistance to the outflow of water. Blood pressure works in exactly the same way, depending on the amount of blood being pumped by the heart and the resistance to the flow of blood. The resistance to blood flow is a function of the width of the arteries, a characteristic that works in the same way the nozzle on the garden hose can constrict and dilate. Arteries that are constricted restrict the flow of blood while increasing the blood pressure. Conversely, if arteries are relaxed and widened, blood flows more easily and blood pressure decreases.

Why We All Must Age-Proof Our Cardiovascular Systems

The famous Framingham Heart Study followed several genera-
tions of residents in the town of Framingham, Massachusetts,
over forty years, taking detailed cardiovascular health assess-
ments on each person every two years. One of the more intriguing findings was that two thirds of participants who started
out with normal blood pressure in their thirties had developed
hypertension. According to the National Institutes of Health,
hypertension plays a role in approximately 700,000 deaths per
year.

Blood pressure is measured in millimeters of mercury (ab-
breviated "mm Hg"), and it is expressed as a fraction—for example, 160/100 or 130/85. As the table below shows, there are
gradations of blood pressure readings; if your blood pressure is
140/90 or higher—the systolic is the top reading and the diastolic is the bottom—your blood pressure is considered high.
Your doctor will tell you that you have hypertension, which
simply put means you have excessive pressure in your arteries.
Even if your blood pressure is in the "high normal" range, you
are at an increased risk for the medical problems associated with
hypertension.

CHECK YOUR BLOOD PRESSURE "RATING"

Blood pressure (mm Hg)	Optimal	Normal	High Normal	Hyper-tension
Systolic (top number)	under 120	120–129	130–139	140 or higher
Diastolic (bottom number)	under 80	80–84	85–89	90 or higher

Silent But Deadly You cannot feel high blood pressure, and this absence of physical symptoms makes hypertension particularly dangerous. Unless you have your blood pressure measured, you will not know whether it is high. Though hypertension does not produce outward signs that damage might be occurring, high blood pressure still may be causing major internal damage by injuring the endothelium—thereby impairing the body's ability to produce its own NO. This scenario gradually leads to inflammation of the arteries, which is followed by atherosclerosis and plaque formation. Hypertension can also enlarge the heart, trigger a heart attack or stroke, and set the stage for kidney failure.

Alarming Facts about Hypertension

According to the findings of the Framingham Heart Study, one half of all people who have first heart attacks, and two thirds of those who have a first stroke, have blood pressure readings above 160/95. If you have hypertension, like 50 million American men and women, you run seven times the risk of having a stroke compared to individuals whose blood pressure is normal.

How NO Fights Hypertension More effective than any other factor in the body, nitric oxide can dilate the smooth muscle of the blood vessels. With this dilation, the vessels can relax and allow blood to flow easily through them—and quite possibly lower the blood pressure.

Amazing But True!

"After only three weeks on NO therapy, my blood pressure was down fifteen points!"

Joe, 45, St. Louis

ATHEROSCLEROSIS

When you are young, the vessels around your heart are flexible, with an internal diameter of about three millimeters, but no one stays young forever. As most people age, the smooth inner walls of their arteries gradually thicken and lose some of their elasticity. At the same time, fatty deposits—or *plaque*—are accumulating on the arterial walls. This process is called *atherosclerosis,* or hardening of the arteries, and when it occurs, it can reduce the diameter of the arteries and impair normal blood flow. Atherosclerosis can cause premature aging and disability. It can impair memory in the middle aged and can foster a form of senile dementia in the elderly. Atherosclerosis is a factor in peripheral artery disease—narrowing of arteries in the legs that leads to inadequate blood flow—especially in smokers in their sixties or older.

Arterial Plaque

You can think of the lining of healthy endothelial cells as being slick like Teflon, while an unhealthy endothelium is sticky like Velcro, causing plaque to attach. The plaque buildup in atherosclerosis is made up not only of fatty substances, including LDL, or "bad" cholesterol, but also waste products from cells, calcium, and a blood-clotting material called fibrin. When this accumulation of "junk" becomes severe in the coronary arteries, it can keep the heart from receiving adequate oxygen from the blood, causing episodes of angina pectoris, or chest pain, which are more likely to occur during exercise or other types of physical exertion when the heart is forced to work harder.

Once plaques become large and brittle, they can crack, rupture, and become dislodged from the arterial walls. As with any other injury, the body may respond by causing blood to clot. When a clot occurs in the arteries, the result can be catastrophic. Clots can jam the vessel passageways, blocking blood flow to the heart and the brain and triggering a heart attack or stroke.

How NO Fights Atherosclerosis Atherosclerosis, like hypertension, is intimately involved with damage to the endothelium, which causes a decline in NO production. For your body to maintain its cardiovascular well-being, it needs to produce healthy amounts of NO. In fact, when your body is manufacturing adequate and even excess nitric oxide, plaque formation and atherosclerosis are much less likely to occur—and may be reversible.

NO More Poor Circulation

"My husband has a circulation problem in one of his legs, and he usually wakes up four or five times a night with pain. Since he has been using NO-boosting supplements, he has not been waking up at all, and he actually sleeps through the night without any discomfort. This has given him incredible energy and a great belief in the healing power of nitric oxide."

Dee, 48, Idaho

HEART ATTACK

A blood clot in your coronary arteries may be only a fraction of an inch thick and weigh less than an ounce, but if it partially or completely deprives your heart of oxygen, it chokes off nourishment that the heart cells need and can cause a heart attack. Your doctor may use a medical term to describe heart attack—*myocardial infarction,* from *myocardial* = heart muscle, and *infarction* = tissue death from oxygen deprivation.

Heart Attack Check List

How would you know if you are having a heart attack? In most cases, one or more of these classic symptoms would be triggered:

- Crushing or uncomfortable pain in the center of the chest, which persists for more than a few minutes, or subsides and then returns. Some people describe the chest pain as pressure or squeezing.

- Pain that radiates down the arms or into the shoulder or neck.

- Chest discomfort that is accompanied by nausea, shortness of breath, or light-headedness.

- Less commonly, heart attack victims may experience nausea, dizziness, unexplained anxiety, depression, or fatigue *without* chest pain.

The Bad Word on Heart Attack

Heart attacks can be triggered by more than blood clots. They may also be caused by excessive plaques in the arteries, or by a temporary but sudden contraction or spasm of the artery called a *vasospasm* that impedes blood flow. Deprived of oxygen, a section of the heart tissue will "starve" and start to die. Serious damage can happen very quickly. According to the American Heart Association, many heart attack patients never make a complete recovery. About half the men and women under sixty-five who have had a heart attack die within eight years of the precipitating event. All the more reason to keep your NO levels high and reduce your chances of ever having a coronary.

The Good Word on Heart Attack

Not every heart attack is fatal. In fact, particularly with prompt care in an emergency room and treatment with so-called "clot-busting drugs," heart attacks are usually survivable. About 1.1 million Americans will have a heart attack this year, and two thirds of them will live to tell about it. Remember, NO can greatly diminish your chances of having a second attack, so even if you are a cardiac patient, you can help yourself.

How NO Fights Heart Attack

By acting to lower blood pressure and cholesterol and improve circulation, NO can offer protection against heart attack.

Reduce Hypertension in NO Time

"My husband has been fighting hypertension for the last year. He was put on blood pressure medication, but this year his blood pressure was even higher, and the medication was increased. He has been under tremendous stress with his job. Well, I put him on a NO-boosting supplement powder the evening of June tenth. Here are some amazing stats:

Before NO Therapy

Date	BP
6/7	150/82
6/8	145/94
6/9	146/96
6/10	141/97

After NO Therapy

6/11	127/87
6/12	121/87

Aren't those results unbelievable? We're a hard-core NO-friendly family from now on!"

Patricia, 53, Boston

STROKE

Although heart attacks strike the heart, and strokes attack the brain, they have more in common than you might think. Both can be triggered by blood clots, although with strokes, these clots settle in the vessels leading to the brain rather than the heart. When that happens, the clots can interfere with normal blood flow and deprive the brain cells of oxygen. The outcome can be brain damage, disability, and even death.

The most common sites for these blood clots are the carotid arteries, which are located on either side of the neck. When the normal production of NO is impaired within the vessel walls, you are much more susceptible to clotting and strokes.

How NO Fights Stroke

Two of NO's critical functions—preventing the formation of blood clots and keeping the arteries free of plaque—work specifically against the occurrence of stroke.

Lifestyle, Lifestyle, Lifestyle

Your doctor may have already talked with you about the risk factors that can raise your chances of developing cardiovascular disease. Though some risk factors are beyond your control, such as a family history of cardiovascular disease, increasing age, and gender, you can influence many others with the lifestyle choices you make, because preventing cardiovascular disease always goes back to the choices you make. Since this book is about preventing and managing cardiovascular disease, some common risk-reduction strategies deserve mention.

Lifestyle Choices You *Must* Make

Stop Smoking If you smoke cigarettes, your risk of cardiovascular disease and a heart attack will at least double. The more cigarettes you smoke per day, the greater your risk. In addition, smoking injures the endothelial cells of your arteries, sabotaging your body's ability to make NO.

Lower Your Blood Cholesterol Level As your cholesterol level climbs, your chances of a heart attack rise as well. Your cholesterol level consists of two readings: the low-density lipoproteins (LDL) or so-called "bad" cholesterol, and the high-density lipoproteins (HDL) or so-called "good" cholesterol. When too much LDL circulates in the blood, it can gradually accumulate on the inner arterial walls and contribute to forming the artery-clogging plaque of atherosclerosis. Clearly LDL is potentially damaging at high enough levels, earning it the "bad" moniker. HDL, on the other hand, is called "good" because it works to remove cholesterol from the arteries and slow the buildup of plaque.

Your LDL reading is the best predictor of your risk of heart attack and stroke, with a higher score indicating a higher risk. LDL cholesterol levels can be broken into the following categories:

LDL CHOLESTEROL LEVELS

Less than 100 mg/dL	Optimal
100 to 129 mg/dL	Near optimal/above optimal
130 to 159 mg/dL	Borderline high
160 to 189 mg/dL	High
190 mg/dL and above	Very high

Another measure of cholesterol that is often used is the cholesterol ratio. Cholesterol ratio is calculated as the total cholesterol (LDL plus HDL) divided by the HDL. For example, a patient with LDL of 150 and HDL of 50 would have a total cholesterol of 200 and a ratio of 200/50 or 4.0. The goal is to have as low a cholesterol ratio as possible, with optimal ratio defined as 3.5. The recommended level is anything below 5.0.

It's Up to You to Control Cholesterol

The LDL cholesterol levels given in the table may be higher than ones you have recently seen, but I stand by them. As this book is going to press there is discussion by established health agencies in the United States about changing these levels. The proposed change is endorsed by the American Heart Association, the American College of Cardiology, and the National Heart, Lung, and Blood Institute, and would result in the optimal value for LDL dropping from 100 mg/dL to 70 mg/dL. The significance of this change is that many more people would be labeled as having high LDL cholesterol and in need of statin drugs.

The proposed changes have created some controversy, and I believe the scientifically prudent thing to recommend is that you know the ranges that have been in effect for several years—the "old" numbers—which are the ones in the table. The proposed changes and your potential need for statin drugs are a matter for you to discuss with your doctor. What I want to communicate most is that you should be doing everything you can to lower your LDL levels naturally.

If you make the dietary and lifestyle changes detailed in my **Say Yes to NO Plan,** your doctor may inform you that your need for statins is either decreased or eliminated. I do not want you simply to depend on drugs and guidelines that change over time to replace your responsibility for your own health. Nature has given you the greatest cardiovascular health wonder drug of them all—nitric oxide—and it is produced right inside your own body. It is up to you to create an environment that lets NO do its job.

NO Therapy Boosts the Effect of Statin Drugs!

With tens of millions of patients taking LDL cholesterol-lowering statin drugs, you might wonder why NO therapy is necessary for lowering cholesterol. The fact is, NO therapy is a natural way of either reducing your need for statins or eliminating the need altogether—without any additional side effects.

Statins do more than just lower cholesterol. Even in low doses they also stimulate NO production in vascular endothelial cells, thereby helping reverse the process of atherosclerosis. Moreover, the NO itself can also help lower cholesterol levels. The overall effect is that statins and NO produce synergistic effects in cardiovascular health.

Our enhanced understanding of the synergy between NO and statins is actually hot off the presses as *NO More Heart Disease* goes to the publisher, as my paper on the subject has just appeared in the prestigious journal *Proceedings of the National Academy of Sciences USA, 2004*. In that very important work, we discovered that combining NO with statin drugs could amplify by several times the effect of the statins in lowering cholesterol. My collaborators in the research went so far as to synthesize a new drug that consists of NO attached to a statin, which is much more effective than each component alone.

I am extremely enthusiastic about the synergy between NO and statin drugs in lowering cholesterol while combating atherosclerosis. The most important message for you to take away from the discussion at this stage is that if you are on statins, you should also undertake NO therapy to amplify your benefits. If you are not on statins, NO therapy may be able to keep you off them. Either way, the benefits of NO therapy in the fight against high cholesterol are too great to ignore. So do not hesitate— start NO therapy immediately.

Control Your Blood Pressure Hypertension makes your heart work harder to keep blood circulating through the body, and it accelerates the wear and tear on your blood vessels. It is therefore imperative that you keep your blood pressure at or below the normal range, which was given earlier as 120/80 to 129/84. A reading of less than 120/80 is most desirable.

Blood pressure is of course a vital sign that does not stay constant with time, but rather it depends on the circumstances surrounding the measurement. Factors such as physical activity, anxiety concerning the visit to a doctor, and even food and drink intake can artificially elevate blood pressure readings. A single blood pressure reading is not an absolute indication of your cardiovascular health. It is best to see your doctor for a complete interpretation of blood pressure measurements.

Keep Your Blood Sugar Under Control High blood sugar levels indicate an excess of glucose (sugar) in the bloodstream, which can result from sickness, overeating, lack of exercise, diabetes, or a number of other adverse factors. High blood sugar is dangerous, because it puts you at increased risk for cardiovascular disease, as well as nerve damage, circulation problems, loss of vision, kidney disease, and sexual dysfunction. A sobering statistic concerning high blood sugar is that the risk of heart disease increases fivefold in diabetic women and twofold in diabetic men.

High blood sugar does have symptoms, including increased thirst, increased hunger, frequent need to urinate, dry and itchy skin, tired or sleepy feeling, blurry vision, nausea, and breathing problems. Blood sugar is measured using a machine called a blood glucose meter, which requires a drop of blood obtained by pricking the skin. It is not a pleasant process to have to continually stick yourself with a needle, so if you do not already have diabetes, you would do well to adopt a NO-producing lifestyle that keeps your blood sugar at normal levels, thus avoiding the need to make these measurements. Target blood sugar levels according to the American Diabetes Association are:

- Between 80 mg/dL and 120 mg/dL before breakfast;
- Between 100 mg/dL and 140 mg/dL during the day and before bed;
- Less than 180 mg/dL one to two hours after a meal.

Do Not Drink Alcohol to Excess One glass of red wine on a daily basis can actually be good for your heart health, because red wine is high in antioxidants that guard your NO supply. If you drink heavily, the process reverses itself, diminishing NO production, which leads to constriction of the vessels and ultimately to a host of cardiovascular conditions—not to mention severe liver damage. Heavy drinking is anything greater than the two drinks a day that define a moderate drinker.

If you are concerned that you cannot help yourself moderate your alcohol consumption, I urge you to join Alcoholics Anonymous. The organization has helped millions and millions of people get clean and sober and stay that way by offering group support and personal understanding of your problem.

Maintain Your Weight at Normal Levels If you are obese, your blood pressure and cholesterol readings are likely to be higher, and your chances of becoming a diabetic may increase as well. The cardiovascular health risks associated with being overweight are well documented. You can hardly turn on the television news without hearing about the latest research study linking obesity and being overweight with poor health. Controlling your weight by eating a healthy, low-fat diet is one of the most basic steps you can take toward improved cardiovascular health. You will learn about such a food program in my **Say Yes to NO** regimen later in the book.

The process of evaluating your weight relative to an ideal weight for your gender, age, and height can be somewhat subjective. In practice, ideal weight is not as simple as looking at a chart, because the standard measure of body weight—the body mass index (BMI)—does not take into account factors like body type. Certainly a highly trained, muscle-bound bodybuilder is going to weigh more for his height than an average person, yet the BMI scale does not allow for these differences in body type and would label the bodybuilder as overweight.

The best general advice I can give here is that if you are at least fifteen to twenty percent heavier than your doctor says you should be, then your excess fat is stressing your heart and blood vessels. Your endothelial NO production is diminished, and your susceptibility to a host of diseases is increased. If you do not know whether you are this far above your doctor-recommended weight, then it is worth your while to see your doctor and find out about your weight and other aspects of your health.

The following charts give some general ranges for ideal body weight in adult men and women. The numbers are statistical averages and not absolutes. Use the charts only as a rough estimate and consult your doctor for a more exact target weight for yourself.

HEIGHT AND WEIGHT TABLE FOR WOMEN

Height Feet Inches	Small Frame	Medium Frame	Large Frame
4' 9"	102–111	109–121	118–131
4' 10"	103–113	111–123	120–134
4' 11"	104–115	113–126	122–137
5' 0"	106–118	115–129	125–140
5' 1"	108–121	118–132	128–143
5' 2"	111–124	121–135	131–147
5' 3"	114–127	124–138	134–151
5' 4"	117–130	127–141	137–155
5' 5"	120–133	130–144	140–159
5' 6"	123–136	133–147	143–163
5' 7"	126–139	136–150	146–167
5' 8"	129–142	139–153	149–170
5' 9"	132–145	142–156	152–173
5' 10"	135–148	145–159	155–176
5' 11"	138–151	148–162	158–179

HEIGHT AND WEIGHT TABLE FOR MEN

Height Feet Inches	Small Frame	Medium Frame	Large Frame
5' 1"	128–134	131–141	138–150
5' 2"	130–136	133–143	140–153
5' 3"	132–138	135–145	142–156

Height Feet Inches	Small Frame	Medium Frame	Large Frame
5' 4"	134–140	137–148	144–160
5' 5"	136–142	139–151	146–164
5' 6"	138–145	142–154	149–168
5' 7"	140–148	145–157	152–172
5' 8"	142–151	148–160	155–176
5' 9"	144–154	151–163	158–180
5' 10"	146–157	154–166	161–184
5' 11"	149–160	157–170	164–188
6' 0"	152–164	160–174	168–192
6' 1"	155–168	164–178	172–197
6' 2"	158–172	167–182	176–202
6' 3"	162–176	171–187	181–207

With an idea of where you fall on the weight charts, I hope your course of action has become clear. I must make one additional point in order to cover the "special cases," which may not be as rare as you think. If you have somehow managed to subsist on mountains of junk food and not end up above your ideal weight range, stop gambling with your health. You have been fortunate, but it would be a good idea to consult a nutritionist and change your eating habits before you do your body even more harm.

Exercise Regularly An extremely effective way of improving your cardiovascular fitness and lowering your risk of heart disease is with aerobic exercise. Exercise can help temper such high-risk conditions as obesity, high blood pressure, high blood sugar, and high cholesterol, thereby reducing the risk of heart attack and stroke. Aerobic activities like walking, running, swimming, and dancing are effective because they "stress" the body's systems for oxygen delivery and energy production. These systems respond to the stress by becoming stronger and healthier. Exercise is a part of my **Say Yes to NO** regimen and will be discussed in more detail later.

Reduce Your Levels of Stress, Anxiety, Loneliness, and Depression This one sounds obvious, yet it is challenging, because these emotional maladies are difficult to quantify. We do know that these emotions can cause blood vessels to constrict through compromised NO production, increasing the likelihood of cardiovascular disease and heart attack. If any of the conditions becomes chronic, then your supply of NO will steadily diminish.

Many sufferers from chronic stress, involuntary solitude, and sadness tend to try to lift their spirits by self-medicating with mood elevators—from tranquilizers to martinis to caffeine. These techniques are detrimental since a temporary high tends to produce an emotional hangover, leaving people even more unhappy than they were before. If you self-medicate, you must discuss it openly with your physician, who may prescribe an antidepressant or recommend that you see a mental health professional. To enjoy optimal health and happiness, which is certainly my goal for you, you must not subject your body and mind to prolonged periods of stress, anxiety, loneliness, and depression.

YOUR PHYSICIAN'S ARSENAL IN THE WAR AGAINST CARDIOVASCULAR DISEASE

If your doctor finds you are already suffering from cardiovascular disease or are a prime candidate, she might recommend a

---

Who Needs Caffeine?

"Since I've been on NO therapy, I find that I sleep so much better. Plus I wake up a lot earlier and am able to feel mentally sharp much faster. I have even skipped coffee recently!"

Barbara, 63, Tucson

---

number of treatments. She may prescribe a statin drug to reduce your cholesterol level or a diuretic or beta-blocker medication for your blood pressure. She may decide you require an angioplasty procedure, in which a balloon-tipped catheter is threaded into an obstructed artery, where it compresses the plaque and opens the artery to restore normal blood flow. You may even be encouraged to undergo coronary artery bypass surgery, in which a vessel from another part of the body is used to reroute the blood flow around clogged vessels in your heart.

All these approaches have a downside as well. Angioplasty, for example, may open the arteries, but those benefits may only be temporary, with a high rate of restenosis or renarrowing, leaving the artery as obstructed as it had been prior to the procedure. Bypass surgery has varying rates of success, depending on the surgeon and the hospital, but a small percentage of patients die from complications during or after this invasive operation.

Amid all these recommendations, you may have noticed a glaring omission. Most doctors overlook nitric oxide, a critical health-promoting strategy that is the focus of this book.

NO TO THE RESCUE

If cardiovascular health is your goal, NO needs to be on the front lines of your heart-healthy program. Many heart attacks and strokes are preventable. You can put a stop to the progression of cardiovascular disease even if you already have it. You are about to take the next step in finding out how.

THE HEART OF THE MATTER

Before we move on, let's review what you have learned in this chapter.

- Almost 62 million Americans have at least one type of cardiovascular disease, including hypertension, coronary heart disease, angina pectoris, and stroke.
- High blood pressure afflicts 50 million men and women.
- A blood pressure reading of 140/90 or more is considered high. Hypertension is a silent disease. It can injure the endothelial cells and cause other physiological damage without any outward signs.
- When your body is producing healthy levels of NO, your risk of plaque formation and atherosclerosis is reduced.
- By lowering the risk of blood clots, NO can decrease the chances of a heart attack or stroke.
- By adopting such lifestyle strategies as reducing blood cholesterol levels and blood pressure, eliminating smoking, and exercising regularly, you can lower your likelihood of cardiovascular disease.

3

THE SCIENCE OF NO:
A CRASH COURSE IN THE INCREDIBLE POWERS
OF THE MIRACLE MOLECULE

NO is one of the simplest molecules in biology, comprised of just two atoms—one atom of nitrogen (N) and one of oxygen (O). Though NO's structure is simple, nitric oxide is now regarded as the most significant molecule in the body, absolutely crucial to your well-being. I am convinced that nitric oxide can age-proof your cardiovascular system, keeping it much fitter than your chronological age would indicate.

For the past two decades, my consuming passion has been the study of this tiny molecule. Year after year—for twelve, fourteen, sixteen hours a day—I have been obsessed with proving its importance. I have concluded that the difference between health and illness is often a function of the level of NO activity in your body. NO can literally be a matter of life and death. Let me tell you why.

HOW YOUNG ARE YOU ON THE INSIDE?

If you are over fifty and have developed an age-related health problem—heart disease or diabetes, for example—you are probably confronting the internal changes that accompany getting older. If you are in your twenties, thirties, or forties, you obviously want to do everything possible to ensure that your heart and your blood vessels remain well-toned for years to come.

However old or young you may be, it is not too late to start on my program to age-proof your inner body.

KEEPING A PULSE ON YOUR HEALTH

It is always important to check with your doctor before beginning a new health regimen. While you are talking to your doctor, be sure to ask for your two most vital health statistics determined during a physical exam: resting pulse rate and blood pressure. Most Americans over the age of forty have no idea of what their pulse and blood pressure measures are and are clueless as to what constitutes high, normal, or low levels. Most of these people know their weight to the ounce but are unaware of numbers that are literally a matter of life and death for them.

The Vital Stats You Must Know

A normal resting pulse rate (the number of times the heart beats per minute) is between 65 and 75. Normal blood pressure is considered to be approximately 125/80—although an article in the September 2003 issue of the *Journal of the American Medical Association* redefined it as 115/75, citing research showing that artery damage can start at this blood pressure level.

NITRIC OXIDE: THE BODY'S NATURAL CARDIOVASCULAR WONDER DRUG

Perhaps you discover from discussing your vital stats with your doctor that you must lower your blood pressure and pulse rates and tone your vessels by reducing constriction in order to keep the blood flowing rhythmically to every cell in your body. The task seems less daunting if you understand the restorative properties of nitric oxide, which is produced in the arteries. NO helps preserve the elasticity of all the vessels, because it is a "signaling molecule" that tells the blood vessels to increase in width or dilate.

Repairing the damage wrought by cardiovascular disease without risky and often ineffective surgery had long been considered impossible. I was awarded the Nobel Prize in Medicine for making that thinking obsolete. Now we know we can reverse cardiovascular impairment naturally—with the body's internally manufactured "wonder drug," nitric oxide.

NO Turns the Tables

"I have three kids under the age of four. Multivitamins helped me keep up with them, but since I've been boosting my NO, the kids can't keep up with me!"

Elaine, 31, New Jersey

Nitric oxide is a powerful signaling molecule present in the cardiovascular and nervous systems as well as throughout the body. NO penetrates membranes and sends specific messages or biological signals that regulate cellular activity and instruct the body to perform certain functions. NO influences the functioning of virtually every bodily organ, including the lungs, liver, kidneys, stomach, genitals, and, of course, the heart.

Among the many vital duties NO performs is its role as a vasodilator, meaning that it helps control blood flow to every part of the body. NO relaxes and enlarges the blood vessels, ensuring that blood can efficiently nourish the heart. NO also works to prevent the formation of blood clots, which are the trigger for strokes and heart attacks, and it regulates blood pressure.

Another key role of NO is to slow the accumulation of atherosclerotic plaque in the blood vessels. You will recall that plaque is an artery-hardening buildup of cholesterol fats in the coronary arteries that can narrow or even block the arteries, thereby reducing the heart's blood supply. My research strongly suggests that by capitalizing on its ability to combat atherosclerotic plaque, nitric oxide therapy can help lower cholesterol by synergistically facilitating the actions of commonly prescribed statin drugs like Lipitor and Mevacor. It stands to reason that NO therapy is not only safe when combined with statins, but also enhancing to the drugs' effects, because one of the important mechanisms of these drugs is to increase and maintain NO production. NO therapy performs the same function, only naturally.

NO is used by the immune system to stave off infectious bacteria, viruses, and parasites, and it even curtails the proliferation of certain types of cancerous cells. In people with moderate to severe diabetes, nitric oxide can prevent many common but serious complications, particularly those associated with impaired blood flow. NO is also crucial to memory function, because the brain uses it to store and retrieve long-term memories, as well as to transmit information. We are currently looking into the major role NO may play in the prevention of Alzheimer's disease.

As an anti-inflammatory, nitric oxide is being studied for its apparent role in reducing the swelling and discomfort of arthritis. NO can also guard against the development of stomach ulcers by maintaining normal blood flow to the mucosal lining of the gastrointestinal system. As a neurotransmitter, NO increases blood flow to the genitals, thus playing an important role in normal sexual functioning. My findings in this area led to the development of the prescription drug Viagra. NO is a powerful antioxidant, deactivating so-called oxygen "free radicals" in the body that can contribute to America's four leading killers: cancer, diabetes, heart disease, and stroke.

It seems that there is no end to the uses of nitric oxide in the body. The number of crucial roles identified for this unique molecule has increased steadily with the growing focus on NO in scientific research. The many uses of NO will be discussed more fully in later chapters, but at this point I wanted you to understand the breadth of its importance to virtually every aspect of body function.

NO PRODUCTION IN THE ENDOTHELIUM

Your own body is the optimal resource for NO production. The manufacture of NO takes place mainly in the endothelium—which you recall is the layer of cells lining the interior surface of the blood vessels. The endothelial tissue, which separates the blood from the smooth muscles of the vessel walls, is extraordinarily thin and fragile. When your endothelium is well nourished, NO is produced at optimal levels and blood flows unimpeded, nurturing the heart along with every other organ. During vigorous exercise, and even during certain routine physiological processes like digestion when more blood is needed, NO makes sure you get it. When the body is at rest, there is less NO, and this cuts back on blood flow.

Because endothelial tissue is just a single cell-layer thick, you might be tempted to believe there is not much margin for error when it comes to keeping it healthy. Although the endothelium is a razor-thin line of demarcation between blood and tissues, it is without doubt one of the body's most tireless workhorses. Industrious, and if anything *over*achieving, endothelial tissue is responsible for keeping our bodies supplied with nitric oxide. With the help of an enzyme called *endothelial NO synthase,* endothelial cells function as the power plant where NO—a renewable resource essential to good health—is manufactured and mobilized.

You need only small amounts of nitric oxide to take advantage of its powerful therapeutic functions, but most people do not produce enough of it to keep their cardiovascular systems functioning smoothly. Underproduction of NO develops when endothelial tissue is damaged by age, an unhealthy lifestyle, illness, a toxic environment, or genetic propensity, and consequently NO production is impaired. Your body becomes vulnerable to virtually every major disease. This book concentrates on cardiovascular disease—specifically, the ways in which a deficiency of nitric oxide can contribute to the illnesses of more than sixty-two million Americans who suffer from elevated blood pressure, atherosclerosis, heart disease, high blood pressure, heart failure, or stroke. If you have deficiencies in NO, we now know they can be offset with an NO-friendly diet, supplement program, and moderate exercise.

SLAMMING THE DOOR ON CARDIOVASCULAR DISEASE

Over a lifetime, the endothelium can become damaged by unhealthy lifestyle and environmental toxins as well as the routine wear and tear accompanying the aging process. When that happens, your inner power plant may produce less NO—or none at all—in the injured regions, leaving you vulnerable to cardiovascular disease.

As resilient as the endothelial cells are, a variety of health conditions can sabotage their well-being, which in turn can impair your body's ability to produce NO. If, for example, you have had moderately to severely high blood pressure for several years, it is probable that the stress on your blood vessels may have already inflicted punishment upon your endothelium, causing damage at such critical sites as the heart and brain. Add to that the other skyrocketing risk factors for endothelial damage—high blood cholesterol levels, elevated blood glucose levels, cigarette smoking, and a steady diet of cholesterol-raising saturated fats—and your endothelium may be taking a most perilous beating.

"I'm a Great Fan of NO!"

"My father passed away from heart disease at the age of fifty-eight. I want to be around a lot longer for my children. I have great faith in NO-boosting supplements along with a good diet and regular exercise routines. I have noticed several positive effects in addition to the long-term health benefits; for one thing, I sleep so much better. Recently, I have started taking the supplements prior to exercising and I find I have better stamina and a lower heart rate during the exercise period. Finally, I have noticed a huge difference in my ability to breathe. I am an allergy sufferer who works outdoors. NO therapy allows me to fill my lungs with fresh air so much more easily than before."

Wayne, 38, Oregon

SHARING THE WEALTH

My life as a researcher has always been challenging and often exhilarating. With the support of graduate students, postdoctoral fellows, visiting scientists, medical fellows, technical assistants, and research collaborators by my side, I would often arrive at five in the morning and work late into the night, driven by the excitement of discovery—those eureka moments—that accompany groundbreaking studies. I am writing *NO More Heart Disease* in the hope and belief that women and men everywhere can reap the priceless health benefits of my more than two decades of research in order to enjoy longer and healthier lives— for themselves and for their loved ones.

THE HEART OF THE MATTER

Before we move on, let's review what you have learned in this chapter:

- Nitric oxide is one of the most significant molecules in the body.

- NO influences the functioning of virtually every human organ, from the heart to the lungs to the stomach.

- NO can relax your blood vessels, reduce your blood pressure, and lower your risk of having a heart attack or stroke.

- Adequate levels of NO may play a role in preventing diabetes complications, Alzheimer's disease, erectile dysfunction, arthritis, infections, and ulcers.

4

NITRIC OXIDE'S ROLE IN THE FOUR ESSENTIAL BODILY PROCESSES

Your body has four essential bodily processes: vascular tone, coagulation, inflammation, and oxidation. Each of these processes can play both a positive and negative role in the body, depending on how they are being applied. In this chapter I explain how nitric oxide therapy can make a life-saving difference to your health by enhancing the positive and eradicating the negative in each of them.

VASCULAR TONE: NO MORE HIGH BLOOD PRESSURE

The Upside of Vascular Tone

What if the smooth muscle tissue of the blood vessels did not have the power to constrict as well as dilate? There would be no way to regulate blood flow. Remember, systolic blood pressure is the force on your arterial walls as your heart beats or contracts to pump out blood. By contrast, the diastolic pressure is the force exerted on the walls as the heart relaxes between beats and fills with blood, preparing to become systolic and start beating. Without sufficient vascular tone, which gives the vessels the power to constrict as well as dilate, our blood would not be able to circulate.

The Downside of Vascular Tone and Constriction

If your blood pressure is high, it indicates that your blood vessels are constricted or there are blockages. If blood does not flow freely, sooner or later the endothelial cells are going to suffer substantial damage. Once NO production is impaired, the risk of heart attack and stroke is greatly increased.

NO to the Rescue

By enhancing the free flow of blood through the body, NO protects the blood vessels' smooth muscle tissue from harmful constriction as it safeguards the health of the endothelium, resulting in NO more high blood pressure.

COAGULATION: NO MORE BLOOD CLOTS

How exactly does nitric oxide prevent clots from developing in your bloodstream? A different process is at work than the one associated with lowering blood pressure. NO draws on its ability to interfere with the leading cause of stroke—the aggregation or coagulation of platelets, tiny disk-shaped bodies made up of cell fragments that are responsible for clotting in the bloodstream.

The Upside of Coagulation

In the right circumstances, clotting is an essential bodily process. If you experience a cut or a puncture on your hand, you not only damage the skin but also the blood vessels underneath it. As you start to bleed, the body's clotting mechanism rushes into action. Platelets immediately congregate and commence adhering to each other, stanching the blood flow by forming a seal to plug the leak and eventually form a scab.

The Downside of Coagulation

If your blood vessel walls have been damaged—perhaps as plaque has accumulated in the walls of your arteries—the platelets may begin to cluster within the bloodstream at the site of the injury. If a *thrombus* or rogue blood clot forms in the area and breaks free, it eventually will block or interfere with blood flow, potentially triggering heart attack or stroke. When a clot occurs in the coronary arteries, it is termed a *coronary thrombosis*; when in a blood vessel leading to or in the brain, it is a *cerebral thrombosis*.

NO to the Rescue

By keeping blood pumping regularly through the vascular system, nitric oxide maintains the vessels and arteries at a prime level of cleanliness. Remember, unhealthy vessels and arteries act like Velcro, attracting and attaching to dangerous foreign matter; while a NO-enhanced vascular network performs like

Teflon, shedding plaque and platelets, inhibiting clots from expanding or from forming in the first place.

INFLAMMATION: NO MORE ATHEROSCLEROSIS

Next, let's focus on another major cardiovascular disease problem: atherosclerosis. The development of atherosclerosis is a gradual, dynamic inflammatory process, taking many years for plaque to develop. NO can intervene early in the process, preventing the thickening of the walls of the arteries and the buildup of fatty material.

The Upside of Inflammation

At controlled levels, inflammation is not always bad. It is an important way your body fights infections. Like a powerful army marching into battle to defend its country, your immune or defense system can mount an attack of such force that it crushes the foreign invaders intent on triggering infections and illness.

The Downside of Inflammation

When this inflammatory process becomes chronic and involves the arteries, it can contribute to the development of conditions like atherosclerosis. The cells that normally function to kill bacteria can turn against you. When inflammation occurs in the blood vessels, it is a process that must be interrupted.

NO to the Rescue

Specifically, here is why sufficient levels of NO are so important in preventing arteriosclerosis. If the endothelial cells on the inner surface of your blood vessels are damaged in any way, other types of cells in the blood, monocytes and leukocytes, can storm through the vessel wall, accumulate, and imbed themselves in the smooth muscle layer. The invasion complete, these cells release chemicals called *inflammatory mediators* that trigger inflammation in the smooth muscle, setting the atherosclerotic process of plaque formation into motion and resulting in blocked blood flow.

Once plaque forms in the arteries, it is much more difficult to undo the damage than to prevent it in the first place. Even so, the strategies in this book can at least stop or slow down the progression. With prevention in mind, nitric oxide can again play a crucial role. After plaques have staked a claim in your arteries, they can grow, become brittle, and break free, lodging in the brain or coronary arteries and setting off a stroke or heart attack.

At the same time, plaque can impair the ability of the endothelium to produce NO, increasing the likelihood that even more plaque will be formed. It is a vicious cycle that can put your life at risk. It is important to prevent plaques altogether with the help of nitric oxide. In fact, there may be no better way of keeping your arteries clean and flexible than to maximize your own production of NO.

It's Never Too Late

Sherry's seventy-two-year-old father from Denver has hardening of the arteries. "He has already lost one leg to the disease and was facing the possibility of losing the other due to constant swelling and pain. After five days on NO therapy, the swelling had been reduced by half and he has hardly any pain!"

OXIDATION: NO MORE OXIDATIVE STRESS

Cardiovascular researchers are focusing a growing amount of attention on so-called "oxidative stress." Of course, oxygen is necessary for life itself, crucial for everything from breathing to keeping your heart beating. When the body uses oxygen, it produces byproducts through the process of oxidation that can be either beneficial or disastrous.

The Upside of Oxidation

Without this process, our cells would not be able to burn glucose, which provides us with energy.

The Downside of Oxidation

The byproducts of oxidation in the body are called oxygen or "free" radicals. Free radicals can create havoc by neutralizing

NO, contributing not only to cardiovascular disease, but also to signs of the aging process from wrinkling of the skin to weakening bones.

Later in the book I discuss oxidative stress in more detail when it comes up in the **Say Yes to NO** regimen. For now, here are some important facts to keep in mind, particularly regarding the role of NO in interrupting this disease process.

To get a clearer image of oxygen free radicals, picture an automobile that burns gasoline for energy, and in the process, generates exhaust filled with harmful pollutants that can turn blue skies to brown. In much the same way, your body relies on oxygen for its energy, but as this energy is being used, it creates its own byproduct of "exhaust"—namely, free radicals.

Although oxidation is associated with routine biochemical processes in the body, these free radicals are sometimes formed in excess. When that happens, this oxidative stress clearly becomes detrimental to your well-being, damaging healthy cells and tissues, including those in the arteries. Free radicals can injure the endothelium. For example, when "bad cholesterol," or LDL, is oxidized, it is chemically altered in ways that allow it to infiltrate the artery walls and do serious damage to the endothelial cells. Though the endothelial cells can repair themselves to some degree, constant oxidative stress can sabotage the opportunity for meaningful self-repair.

NO to the Rescue

NO can minimize the oxidative stress that contributes to cardiovascular disease. There is a complicating factor but certainly not an insurmountable one. When free radicals are present in high numbers, they try to overpower and disarm the NO produced by your body before it can take control of the situation. When your body is in a state of oxidative stress, you may have much less NO than normal. Antioxidants can help. Antioxidants act like scavengers in the body, searching for free radicals and neutralizing them before they can cause much damage. Many of the supplements in my **Say Yes to NO Plan** are antioxidants that can destroy free radicals in the blood vessels and throughout the body.

It's Better to Be Safe . . .

Ethan, a high-powered twenty-nine-year-old stock broker from Chicago, takes good care of himself, including working out five days a week. He is in great shape but still has health concerns, because his family on both sides has a history of cardiovascular problems. In fact, his father, Gerald, has just suffered a mild heart attack at the relatively young age of fifty-five. Ethan has been following the nitric oxide story, beginning with the Nobel Prize, and is intrigued. Searching the Web, he found a supplement specifically formulated to increase the body's production of NO and ordered one of them for his dad. The results were astonishing.

In a matter of weeks, Gerald's blood pressure was approaching normal as was his cholesterol level. He was also sleeping better and recovering remarkably quickly from the heart attack. "I will never go off this stuff," Gerald announces. "It's literally life-saving!"

Following in his father's footsteps, Ethan has begun taking the supplements as a preventive measure. He says that after a couple of months on the regimen, he has twice the energy he used to have and can accomplish more in half the time than he could before he became a NO man!

THE NO WORKSTATIONS: BEYOND THE ENDOTHELIUM

At the same time that the vascular endothelial cells are manufacturing nitric oxide, other workstations in the body are making NO as well. While the endothelium is the primary factory for nitric oxide, certain types of nerve cells can also produce NO. For example, when nerves in the erectile tissue of the penis are stimulated, they activate the enzyme *neuronal NO synthase* that immediately produces NO, which then enters the smooth muscle of the penis, causing it to relax. As this relaxation takes place, the penis can accommodate more blood, which in turn produces an erection. My research in this area laid the foundation for the development of the drug Viagra.

Nitric oxide is also produced by nerve cells in the brain and the lungs. When nerves in the lungs release NO, the presence of this molecule can cause dilation of the airways, called bronchodilation. In the brain, NO is manufactured in regions associated with improving memory and learning, as well as influencing and modifying our behavior.

NO is produced in one other important site: the white blood cells. These cells come in various sizes and shapes, and they are the backbone of the body's immune system. Present in numbers exceeding one billion in the typical man or woman, this massive army of cells can destroy most external invaders, from bacteria to viruses to parasites. As part of this defense system, the white blood cells produce nitric oxide in such large quantities that the NO can help overpower the attacking microorganisms.

NO can positively influence many other diseases and disorders—from cancer to digestive problems, from tuberculosis to learning disorders. Since NO acts as a signal molecule throughout the nervous system, it communicates messages that affect the heart, lungs, kidneys, stomach, brain, and genitals, among other organs. In fact, there may be no disease process in the body in which nitric oxide does not have a protective role. Though NO has a very short lifespan, more NO is constantly being produced in a body with healthy endothelial cells.

In the chapters that follow, I will challenge you to adopt the simple but proven lifestyle modifications that can transform your health. The dietary changes, supplements, and exercise regimen are uncomplicated, but they will significantly boost your body's natural production of NO in a safe and medically sound manner.

Our increasing understanding of NO, which has resulted in my **Say Yes to NO** program, is one of the most important advances in medicine in recent years. You now have the opportunity to take advantage of all that we have learned about it, and your body will reap the benefits.

THE HEART OF THE MATTER

Before we move on, let's sum up what you have learned in this chapter:

- The endothelial cells are workhorses in the cardiovascular system, manufacturing the NO that guards against many common diseases. By controlling blood flow, they can help regulate blood pressure.

- Once plaque forms in the arteries, it is difficult to undo the damage. Thus, prevention is key, and NO can play an important role in keeping plaques at bay.

- By interfering with platelet aggregation, NO minimizes the risk of strokes.

- "Oxidative stress" can contribute to cardiovascular disease, but the damage caused by oxygen radicals can be reduced with the proper choice of supplements.

- You can restore the functioning of injured endothelial cells by taking select amino acid and antioxidant supplements that stimulate NO production.

- NO is not only produced by the endothelial cells in the blood vessels, but also by nerve cells and white blood cells.

5

SAY YES TO NO: MY THREE-PART PROGRAM FOR CARDIOVASCULAR AGE-PROOFING — AN OVERVIEW

My three-part **Say Yes to NO** program is designed for maximal cellular nutrition. I have created a system of cellular nourishment based on the principle of synergy—in which several elements working together produce far greater results than the sum of the individual elements. As you will see, synergy also means that when certain elements are taken together, they increase each other's effectiveness.

In order to get a measurable benefit from your nitric oxide therapy, it is critical that any NO-boosting supplements you purchase be in adherence with the **Say Yes to NO** program. You must be sure that you are taking the appropriate dosages of the nutrients I recommend, and that you do not omit any of the supplements. The program's effectiveness is based upon the synergistic combination of the amino acids L-arginine and L-citrulline, as well as four key antioxidants. Most products available on the market claiming to boost your NO are effectively just L-arginine—in insufficient doses—which do not deliver the cardiovascular health results that are available from the **Say Yes to NO** program. Be vigilant—it will be worth the effort.

Bright-Eyed and Bushy-Tailed

Caroline, a thirty-two-year-old from San Francisco, feels that a NO-boosting supplement package lifted the fog from her mornings. "To give you an idea of what I was like before beginning nitric oxide supplementation—I wore pajamas with the saying 'I'm allergic to mornings.' It used to take me an hour or more to start really functioning. Now I fall asleep fast, sleep through the night, and have been getting up before the alarm goes off. Instead of waking up groggy, I wake up alert and in a good mood. And I'm able to pack as many things into my day as I did when I was eighteen!"

BUILDING THE NO POWERHOUSE

Here is how synergy works in my NO-boosting regimen:

Nutraceutical supplements—natural bioactive compounds with health promoting or medicinal qualities—are powerful on their own, but when they are taken together, they increase each other's NO-boosting efficiency more than if you added them up separately. In the NO-boosting regimen, the nutraceutical supplements are a mix of specific amino acids and antioxidants. I firmly believe that whether you have developed cardiovascular problems or simply want to prevent them, a daily supplement package is necessary.

Certain *functional foods,* including red meat, fish, olive oil, nuts, and pomegranate juice, are known to enhance the body's ability to produce nitric oxide. Functional foods refer to food products formulated with naturally occurring compounds to provide a health benefit or lower the risk of disease. Unfortunately in the case of NO, you would have to eat one hefty steak after another all three meals a day to maintain a beneficial level of nitric oxide. If you want to safeguard your cardiovascular health, you should design your meals around NO-friendly foods, but diet alone will not get your NO factory functioning at full capacity.

During *exercise,* the body produces nitric oxide at an elevated rate. There is really no downside to exercise, but unless you intend to be at the gym 24/7, exercise alone will not provide you with the amount of NO you need. Proper diet combined with exercise increases the production of nitric oxide at a rate greater than that of each element separately. In fact, these two components of the NO-boosting regimen may even heighten each other's effectiveness . . . but they do not raise the production of nitric oxide to the level our bodies require for optimal health.

The Big Payoff

If you combine a NO-friendly diet, moderate exercise, and the proper amino acids and antioxidants, your body will become a NO-producing powerhouse, keeping endothelial cells well nourished and blood vessels relaxed, which can lower your blood pressure and cholesterol, discourage the formation of plaques, ensure blood flow, and reduce the inflammation which can lead to atherosclerosis—often in as little as two weeks.

What a Way to Go!

"I'm a frequent international traveler," writes Susan, fifty-one, from Miami, "and jet lag had become a part of my life—until I began my nitric oxide regimen. Shortly after I started, I noticed that my frequent jet lag was suddenly less frequent and less severe. I take my NO-boosting supplement package each evening, whether I'm at home or traveling. As a result, I'm able to sleep through the night and awake refreshed, no matter where I am or what time it is in my head."

SAY YES TO NO-BOOSTING SUPPLEMENTS

In the program I will be asking you to consume a specially designed blend of nutraceutical cellular nutrients that includes the following:

- *L-arginine* is a naturally produced protein building block called an *amino acid*. L-arginine enhances blood flow and improves the activity of the endothelial cells because it is converted to NO in the body. Although L-arginine is found in some foods (red meat, fish, chicken, beans, soy, nuts), you cannot normally consume sufficient amounts in your diet from meals alone. So I will be recommending that you take L-arginine supplements each day.

- A second amino acid, *L-citrulline,* is closely related to L-arginine and is found in many of the same protein-

rich foods and also in melons. In your body, L-citrulline is converted into L-arginine, which in turn increases the production of NO. I will also be
recommending that you take L-citrulline in supplement form.

- Certain key vitamins—including *Vitamins C, E, and
  folic acid*—act as antioxidants in the body, preserving
  your supply of nitric oxide. These vitamins can combat the disease-promoting process called "oxidation,"
  which inactivates NO, reduces its concentrations in the
  body, and damages the endothelial cells. Taking antioxidant supplements can make a difference. At the
  dosage levels that I will advocate, they will block the
  oxidation process, promote healing of the endothelial
  lining, and protect the NO that your body produces.

- *Alpha lipoic acid* is still another important natural
  source of antioxidants—which may indeed have a
  synergistic effect with the above nutrients. This supplement is produced in the body, and its primary role
  is in cellular energy production. Any excess alpha
  lipoic acid not required for energy production serves
  as an antioxidant, where it helps to remove an unusually large number of cell-damaging free radicals.

Lower Blood Pressure—in Half an Hour!

At Hannover Medical School in Germany, ten healthy
men were given intravenous L-arginine (a 30-gram dose
administered over thirty minutes). Patients experienced
not only a decrease in their blood pressure readings, with
the declines more pronounced in diastolic than systolic

pressures, but there was also a 33 percent reduction in the clumping or aggregation of their blood platelets. NO levels measured in the urine increased as well (the so-called NO_3—a metabolite or derivative of NO—rose 65 percent following the infusion of L-arginine).

PROTEIN POWER

A little background on protein will help you better understand the importance of amino acids such as L-arginine. Protein is a complex organic substance found in many foods. It is crucial for the maintenance of the body's tissue, the formation of muscles and organs, wound healing, energy, and the regulation of many physiological processes, including the movement of oxygen and nutrients throughout the body.

Protein is the body's major building material. When you eat protein-rich foods like red meat, fish, poultry, tofu, egg whites, and nuts, the digestive enzymes in the small intestine break the protein down into its simplest forms, which are the many compounds called amino acids. L-arginine is one of them. L-citrulline is another.

How L-Arginine = NO

After L-arginine is consumed in foods and in supplements, it makes its way into the bloodstream and circulates throughout the body. As it enters the endothelial cells that line the smooth muscle walls of the blood vessels, an enzymatic reaction occurs that converts L-arginine to NO. As the levels of L-arginine rise in the body, so does your production of NO, which in turn can have a dramatic and positive effect on your cardiovascular health.

Your Priceless Recyling Pathway: L-Arginine Meets L-Citrulline

When L-arginine is synergized with L-citrulline, nitric oxide output is increased. There is a unique relationship between L-arginine and L-citrulline. For many years, scientists believed that L-arginine was not manufactured in the body and had to be obtained from functional foods and nutraceuticals. More recently, scientists have discovered that our bodies can, in fact, manufacture L-arginine through a synergistic interaction with L-citrulline, known as the L-citrulline/L-arginine recycling pathway. L-arginine present in the cells is converted into NO, creating the byproduct L-citrulline in the process. This L-citrulline byproduct, along with any additional L-citrulline that has been introduced by means of food intake or supplements, can be converted back into L-arginine—which is then converted into more NO. This "turbo-charging" effect of the L-citrulline/L-arginine recycling pathway can substantially increase NO production.

I want to be clear that it is extremely important for you to use the right combination that includes L-citrulline along with L-arginine in your supplement routine. There are a number of supplement packages on the market that are billed as NO-boosters but which do not contain L-citrulline. If you choose such a supplement package, you will be missing out on the benefits you can gain from NO therapy. Be sure to check labels carefully on any packaged supplement to verify that the ingredients and dosages are in line with my prescriptions in the next chapter.

Weighing the Evidence

Can L-arginine and L-citrulline converted to NO restore and protect your cardiovascular health? Ongoing research is now answering that question in the affirmative, and the evidence continues to be increasingly persuasive. On an anecdotal level, many people have written me that, after just two to three weeks on L-arginine supplements, they have witnessed a sharp decline in their blood pressure readings. In some cases the decline was so dramatic that pressure actually normalized, something that prescription blood pressure medications are not always successful in doing.

L-Arginine in Circulation

In another study at Hannover Medical School, scientists examined the effects of L-arginine on peripheral artery disease, which involves the narrowing of blood vessels to the leg arteries, leading to symptoms like severe pain in the calf muscles during walking (a condition called "intermittent claudication"). The investigators evaluated thirty-nine patients with intermittent claudication, giving them either two daily infusions of L-arginine (8 grams each), prostaglandin E1 (a vasodilator), or no treatment for three weeks. Those individuals receiving L-arginine experienced greater improvement in their pain-free walking dis-

---

> tance and their absolute walking distance than those on
> prostaglandins, while there was no significant change
> in the control patients. L-arginine also improved the ves-
> sel dilation in the thighs associated with endothelial
> function, while prostaglandin produced no such im-
> provement. The researchers concluded, "Restoring NO
> formation and endothelium-dependent vasodilation by
> L-arginine improves the clinical symptoms of intermittent
> claudication in patients with peripheral arterial occlusive
> disease."

In particular, the most impressive declines with L-arginine have been seen in the diastolic pressure—the bottom number of the blood pressure fraction—which may be related to the dilation of blood vessels associated with L-arginine-related increases in NO levels.

L-arginine and L-citrulline are heavyweight ingredients in my formula for NO potency—especially when they are synergized with our second silver bullet: antioxidants.

OXYGEN: YOUR FRIEND *AND* FOE

Oxygen is key to your existence. You inhale and exhale thousands of times a day, providing yourself with about 2,600 gallons of life-sustaining air during every twenty-four hours. Without it, you could not survive for more than a few minutes.

In one of nature's greatest paradoxes, oxygen has a negative aspect—*oxidation,* which has been discussed in the previous chapter. Oxygen keeps you alive, but it can sabotage your wellness with *oxidative stress,* which not only radically reduces the levels of nitric oxide in your body but in time causes NO to become inactive. Oxidative stress is caused when oxygen molecules become unstable, leading to chaos in your body.

Invasion of the Free Radicals

For decades, researchers studying oxidative stress believed that derivatives of oxygen could cause or contribute to many diseases, but there was little or no evidence to support that hypothesis. Now we have proof.

In an oxygen atom, the particles called electrons rotate around the atom's nucleus in pairs, like planets orbiting around the sun. When these electrons remain paired, the oxygen atom stays stable. When an electron breaks free, causing the atom to be suddenly short an electron, the molecule destabilizes, forming *oxygen radicals* or *free radicals*. Free radicals will do anything to stabilize. Attempting to return to normal, they hijack electrons from any other compounds they can plunder within the cells. As this occurs, nearby cell structures are destroyed, triggering an ominous chain reaction of cell damage that creates even more free radicals. More cells are injured and killed in a vicious cycle. Stability becomes a thing of the past. Tissues can become damaged, and entire physiological systems can break down.

The Free Radicals Around You

Free radicals can form not only through normal biochemical processes, but also through exposure to many environmental chemicals. If you smoke cigarettes, for example, substances in the smoke can trigger the creation of free radicals that injure the lining of the lungs.

Other environmental pollutants, including chemicals in the air and water and pesticides in food, can cause oxidative stress and result in substantial cellular damage. The same is true with excessive exercise, radiation from X-rays, and ultraviolet light from the sun or a sun lamp. Even emotional stress—at high levels for extended periods of time—can spark the production of free radicals. My **Say Yes to NO Plan** is targeted specifically to attack free radicals before they deactivate nitric oxide molecules.

Good Cop, Bad Cop: Free Radicals' Contradictory Roles

For years, scientists had difficulty identifying all the mechanisms involved in the damage associated with free radicals. Today, studies in my own lab and in many others have shown that free radicals cause much of their damage by radically depressing your body's levels of NO. Despite this destructive role of free radicals, there is reason to be encouraged, because they perform an equally important part in the NO-production cycle.

NO has a lifespan of only a fraction of a second. If it existed for much longer, it would begin to take a devastating toll on your physical well-being. Though NO may be able to lower your blood pressure more effectively than any prescription medication your doctor could ever recommend, it would probably lower your pressure to dangerous, even life-threatening levels if not properly regulated. That is how free radicals play a positive role. Free radicals essentially destroy the NO that has already done its job as a signaling molecule, keeping your NO at optimal levels.

It is a delicate balance. Your body needs free radicals to inhibit the action of nitric oxide, preventing the body from being overrun by NO. At the same time, you need a plentiful amount of NO to ensure your good health. When your body is unable to achieve the right balance, you can get NO production back on track with my **Say Yes to NO** regimen.

The Antioxidants Strike Back!

Thanks to our own internal antioxidants—an extraordinary group of vitamins and other natural substances—many free radicals are destroyed before they can cause serious damage. Because they neutralize free radicals, antioxidants are considered nitric oxide's watchdogs, stabilizing and protecting NO during its brief existence—even extending its life. Dozens, perhaps hundreds of these endogenous antioxidants are produced naturally by cells in the body. Hence, the antioxidants I prescribe in my program play a critical role, not only in helping your body produce more NO, but also in allowing it to make constructive use of the NO that it does produce.

Nitric oxide is a potent antioxidant in its own right, able to fend off destructive free radicals. Among all the endogenous antioxidants, NO is the most important since it seeks out, reacts with, and neutralizes free radicals wherever it can find them. Nitric oxide is one thousand times more powerful than any other natural antioxidant in the body.

When it performs its antioxidant role, NO acts as an anti-inflammatory agent, interacting with enzymes and genes to minimize many inflammatory processes. It is constantly waging an internal war with disease-promoting chemicals in the body, prevailing more often than not.

When your levels of naturally occurring NO are not sufficient to combat free radicals, backup help from antioxidant supplements—especially when synergized with L-arginine and L-citrulline—can give your body the protection it needs. We will examine amino acids and antioxidants in a chapter devoted exclusively to them. For this discussion, recognizing antioxidants as key components in any comprehensive NO-boosting regimen is sufficient.

With the help of vitamin C, vitamin E, folic acid, and alpha lipoic acid, synergized with L-arginine and L-citrulline, you will substantially limit the toxic effects of oxidation while bolstering its NO-friendly functions. You will encourage your endothelial cells to begin repairing themselves. You will increase your production of NO. All of this contributes to being healthy—and staying healthy.

Vitamin E and Endurance

An intriguing study of the effect of vitamin E on physical performance was published in the *International Journal of Vitamin and Nutrition Research* in 1988. As part of this research, a group of high-altitude mountain climbers were given either 200 IU of vitamin E twice a day or a placebo, while participating in a ten-week expedition. The group taking vitamin E experienced improved physical performance and greater cell protection than the placebo group, due to lower levels of free radicals in the body.

The second crucial element of **Say Yes to NO** is a balanced nutritional program that emphasizes L-arginine and L-citrulline, along with antioxidants to shore up your body's NO production.

SAY YES TO NO-BOOSTING NUTRITION

I find it interesting that so many people can exhibit common sense in most areas of their lives, yet when it comes to food they seem to become totally irrational. There is a prevailing attitude, perpetuated in large part by advertisers, that the purpose of food is flavor and comfort. Many people thus choose to consume foods that are flavorful and satisfying in the moment, totally disregarding the true needs of their bodies. The food we eat is not just recreation, it is the essential fuel that keeps our bodies running. And even more so than with an automobile, the particular grade of fuel we choose has an enormous effect on the performance of our bodies.

An important part of feeding your body the right fuel is being sure to include sufficient amounts of such NO-producing functional foods as seafood and blueberries, which specifically work to enhance your body's production of nitric oxide. As with most things in life, the key to maintaining your heart health through functional foods—especially when they are synergized with the nutraceuticals I recommend—is moderation.

Although nutraceuticals are critical to the production of nitric oxide, they are not magic. Even if you take them conscientiously, you cannot expect to eat a twelve-ounce steak seven nights a week without battering and bruising your arteries and endothelial cells. L-arginine, vitamins C and E, folic acid, and alpha lipoic acid will not protect you from that kind of high-fat, high-cholesterol dietary assault. If you eat excessive amounts of any food, even if it is healthy, you are going to gain weight and damage your health. A key requisite of dietary moderation is portion control. The **Say Yes to NO Plan** will not require you to become a fanatic about what you prepare in your kitchen and serve at the dining room table.

In Chapter 7, I will detail some important but moderate dietary guidelines—not a rigid day-by-day, meal-by-meal plan, but a general approach to eating, with *every* component proven to be NO-friendly. I will share with you some of my dietary rules, along with tips on being NO-conscious without living like a Zen monk. I want you to enjoy your meals—within reason. That is why the organizing principle of my nutritional guidelines is "good things in moderation." I will talk more about the specifics of NO-boosting foods in Chapter 7.

WITH THIS KIND OF POSITIVE REINFORCEMENT, IT'S EASY TO CHANGE

Making NO-boosting lifestyle adjustments and sticking with them is not so hard to do, because you start to feel better almost immediately. Many people on **Say Yes to NO** have seen their blood pressure and cholesterol readings sharply decline in a couple of weeks and report they are experiencing an enhanced sense of energy and well-being. We have seen how NO-boosting nutraceuticals, synergized with complementary functional foods, ratchet up the body's production of nitric oxide. There is one more factor in the equation—exercise.

SAY YES TO NO-BOOSTING FITNESS

Since physical activity accelerates blood flow, elevates levels of the enzyme NO synthase that produces NO, and increases the amount of nitric oxide in the body, I have made exercise a major component of the **Say Yes to NO Plan**. In fact, exercise is the leading strategy for promoting consistent and continuous production of NO by the vascular endothelial cells. You may be happy to hear that you do not need to push yourself to the brink of exhaustion to enjoy the benefits of physical activity. In fact, I recommend adopting a moderate exercise program of about twenty minutes, three days a week, which virtually everyone can manage, from the most sedentary individuals to the fittest athletes.

NO More Excuses!

I have heard all the rationalizations for staying sedentary— I'm too old, too busy, I can't afford it, I don't have the time. I accept none of these lame excuses. First off, you are never too old to exercise. A Tufts University study reports that even people in their nineties can restore muscle mass. Secondly, if you are too busy to make time for moderate exercise, you are probably under a lot of stress, most likely do not pay attention to what you eat, and maybe even drink excessively to relieve the pressure. I am sure you will get another promotion—a few months before your heart attack. For people who intend to enjoy long, productive lives, working out is not voluntary; it is mandatory. If you are not interested in saving your life, you should do it for your loved ones. As far as the cost of a gym membership is concerned, I do not buy that excuse either. You do not have to join a gym. Walk. Or jog. Or ride a bicycle. There are plenty of ways to boost NO production through exercise without spending a lot of money.

Twenty Minutes to NO

If you are exercising for the first time, you need to make only a moderate—there's that word again—commitment. I recommend you begin working out for twenty minutes, three times a week. That schedule is often enough to keep your NO production way up. The benefits will last after you have finished your exercise. In Chapter 8, I will explain how exercise affects blood pressure, cholesterol, and arterial plaque. You must make exercise part of your life right now.

Getting the Edge Back with NO!

"I was starting from ground zero with my running," reports Dan, a forty-five-year-old San Diego resident and a big fan of nitric oxide therapy. "This year, after I'd begun using NO-boosting nutraceuticals and functional foods, it took me only three weeks to start clocking the same running times that took me eight weeks last year. And after I run, my pulse goes back to normal much more quickly. My recovery time has really improved! NO therapy has given me back the edge I had in my thirties."

Customizing Your Workout

Only you can design an exercise regimen that will not bore you. In the chapter on exercise I will provide you with a list of possibilities, ranging from walking to dancing. Study it and decide what activities or series of activities have the most appeal to you. Your chances of sticking with the program are vastly improved if you enjoy what you are doing.

I will also provide you with pointers that will help you get the most from NO-boosting fitness. You will become passionate about the natural high you feel when the NO starts pumping through your body.

Now you have the basics of **Say Yes to NO.** I advise you to get with the program as soon as possible. The sooner you begin, the sooner you will start realizing the benefits. This NO-boosting synergy of nutraceuticals, functional foods, and exercise will make you feel better, look better, and function better—as it protects you from cardiovascular disease.

THE HEART OF THE MATTER

Before we move on, let's review what you have learned in this chapter.

- L-arginine is an amino acid manufactured to some degree in the body, with the help of another amino acid, L-citrulline.
- L-arginine is capable of increasing the body's levels of nitric oxide, and in turn, improving cardiovascular

health, by lowering total and LDL cholesterol levels and reducing platelet aggregation.

- Even though oxygen is essential to life, it is involved in a process called oxidation that can make nitric oxide inactive.

- Free radicals (also called oxygen radicals) are produced by oxidative stress. They are unstable molecules that can cause damage to healthy cells and tissue, alter DNA and genetic material, and potentially impair entire physical systems, leading to serious disease.

- Certain vitamins, called antioxidants, can interfere with oxidative stress and optimize your internal chemical balance.

- The acceleration of blood that occurs during exercise can stimulate production of the enzyme NO synthase, which is important to the body's production of NO.

6

SAY YES TO NO-BOOSTING SUPPLEMENTS

Now that you have mastered the basic facts about amino acids and antioxidants, I will review the components of my NO-boosting nutraceutical package in terms of efficacy and dosage as well as the results of some remarkable studies on supplement-induced, intensified NO production.

Let's begin by reviewing some basic facts about the amazing amino acids L-arginine and L-citrulline.

THE STORY OF L-ARGININE

It all started in 1980, when Dr. Robert Furchgott discovered that the endothelial tissue lining the walls of blood vessels manufactured a substance that kept the vessels smooth and dilated in a healthy person. Next, scientists found that high cholesterol worked against the endothelium's ability to relax the vessels. We had become convinced that nitric oxide was the relaxation mechanism, but we were not sure how it worked. In 1988, a British scientist, Salvador Moncada, identified the substance that converts to NO in the endothelium—an amino acid called L-arginine. Did that mean an infusion of L-arginine could encourage NO production in the endothelium? If it could, would it help lower cholesterol and keep the vessels clean and smooth, discouraging cardiovascular disease? Subsequently, scientists, including cardiologist John P. Cooke of the Stanford School of Medicine, achieved positive results in trials on human beings, confirming the cardiovascular benefits of L-arginine.

WHAT L-ARGININE AND L-CITRULLINE CAN DO FOR YOUR HEALTH

L-arginine and L-citrulline play critical roles in the body's production of NO. NO is critical to your cardiovascular wellness, and L-argnine, which is enhanced by L-citrulline, is an important component in stimulating your body's production of nitric oxide. L-citrulline, as we know, is an amino acid that is utilized by the vascular endothelial cells and converted into L-arginine, thereby providing even more "fuel" to produce nitric oxide.

L-Arginine: Essential, Nonessential—or Something Else?

Your body needs not only L-arginine and L-citrulline but a broad range of amino acids to maintain good health. Some of them are manufactured within the body's cells and for that reason, they are called *nonessential* amino acids. By contrast, *essential* amino acids are not produced by the body and must be acquired through diet and supplements.

For many years, L-arginine and L-citrulline were categorized as essential amino acids, based on the understanding that they were not manufactured in the body and had to be obtained externally. Recently scientists have discovered that the body can, in fact, manufacture some L-arginine with the help of the other NO-boosting amino acid, L-citrulline, which is formed inside the cells of the body, where it is converted into L-arginine.

You make some L-arginine and L-citrulline of your own, but your body can use more of these amino acids for optimal health. For that reason, L-arginine and L-citrulline are often described as *semi-essential* amino acids.

THE NUTRACEUTICAL ADVANTAGE

Since amino acids are the building blocks of protein, it should come as no surprise that the best sources of dietary L–arginine and L-citrulline are protein-rich foods such as red meat, chicken, and fish. However, focusing on dietary consumption of L-arginine and L-citrulline can be risky, because many of the food sources of these amino acids contain excess saturated fat. A safer strategy for boosting intake is the addition of supplements, which provide all the benefits of L-arginine and L-citrulline, without the drawbacks of high fat meals.

L-Arginine Reverses Endothelial Dysfunction

At the Mayo Clinic in 1999, a six-month-long study was designed to examine whether supplements of L-arginine could reverse endothelial dysfunction in people with coronary artery disease. Twenty-six patients participated in the study, and received either oral L-arginine supplements (3 grams a day) or placebo. After six months, the endothelial function and blood flow throughout the coronary vessels improved in the supplement group, as did the symptoms of coronary artery disease in these patients.

SETTING L-ARGININE DOSAGE GOALS

Whether your L-arginine comes from diet or supplements, only a portion of it will become "bioavailable," making its way through the digestive system, into the bloodstream and then into the cells. The rest is eliminated or excreted from the body in the urine or feces. Probably much less than half of the L-arginine you consume will ever travel along the proper pathways and enter the cells where it can be converted to NO. For that reason, I recommend that you take a high dose of supplemental L-arginine to ensure that adequate amounts make their way into the endothelial cells, leading to increases in your levels of your bodily produced nitric oxide.

Most people take in between 1 and 2 grams a day of dietary L-arginine, although it may be a little higher for people who consume plenty of red meat. With increases in NO production as a goal, my recommendation is to try to ingest as much L-arginine in your diet as possible without consuming red meat in excess, and then supplement that intake with L-arginine in powder or pill form.

There are two options for receiving the optimal supplemental dose:

L-ARGININE SUPPLEMENT DOSAGE

Option 1: Once a day, before bedtime:	4–6 grams a day (4–6 1000 mg L-arginine tablets)
Option 2: Twice a day, in the morning and before bedtime:	2–3 grams in the morning (2–3 1000 mg L-arginine tablets) 2–3 grams before bedtime (2–3 1000 mg L-arginine tablets)

There are some NO-producing supplement packages sold on the market that contain significantly less L-arginine than my recommended 4 to 6 grams. If you are looking to buy a product of this type, be very aware of the levels of L-arginine. My research shows that if you are receiving less than four grams a day in supplement form, the increase in NO production is virtually negligible. Your L-arginine dosage is an "all or nothing" proposition. Be sure that your supplement provides you with at least 4 grams of L-arginine a day.

It is best to take L-arginine just before retiring for the night. Our vascular endothelial cells produce less NO during sleep than when we are awake and moving around. Body movement stimulates NO production. Most heart attacks occur at night, during the early morning hours, when our endothelial cells produce only minimal amounts of nitric oxide.

L-Arginine and Cardiac Output

In research conducted by Tokyo's Keio University School of Medicine in 1992, patients were given intravenous doses of L-arginine that produced rapid lowering in blood pressure as well as marked increases in the volume of blood the heart pumps per beat, called the cardiac output. The investigators concluded "our results provide evidence for the first time that systemically administered L-arginine releases NO in man."

Results of further L-arginine studies are discussed at the end of this section.

L-ARGININE: WORKING WONDERS WITHOUT A DOWNSIDE

If you choose to take my recommended dose of L-arginine, you can expect no side effects. L-arginine is a very safe amino acid and can be taken at the 4 to 6 grams dose without any worry about toxicity. In fact, doses at much higher levels have caused no serious adverse effects in clinical trials.

In one study a patient did develop a recurrence of a cold sore (a type of herpes simplex) on the lips with high-dose L-arginine (9 grams a day), but it disappeared once the individual went off the amino acid. There is some discussion among patients and even some physicians of L-arginine causing herpes outbreaks. The likely reason for this misinformation is that in the herpes virus duplication process, proteins are produced that are rich in L-arginine. However, the fact that L-arginine is a product of the herpes duplication process does not mandate the conclusion that L-arginine causes herpes. In fact, I know of no studies that demonstrate an increase in herpes outbreaks in large populations of patients as a result of L-arginine intake. In the unlikely event that you begin taking L-arginine and do experience a herpes outbreak, you may want to discontinue L-arginine use and the outbreak should subside within a week or so.

There have been no additional reports of side effects or adverse effects linked to L-arginine. No side effects have been reported in the medical literature. Even so, it is always a good idea to check with your physician before taking any supplement or drug; he or she knows your medical history better than anyone.

L-CITRULLINE DOSAGE GOALS

There is very little published information on L-citrulline as a dietary supplement, but I suspect that more data will become available as scientists better recognize that NO can be produced indirectly from L-citrulline after conversion to L-arginine. You must remember that L-citrulline combines with L-arginine to create a synergistic effect, and it is therefore critical for you to include L-citrulline in your supplement program. My recommended daily supplemental dose of L-citrulline is:

L-CITRULLINE SUPPLEMENT DOSAGE

Once a day, before bedtime:	200–1000 mg

L-citrulline supplements have historically been a challenge to find, but recently the number of places they can be found in pill or powder form on the Internet has increased considerably. And do not forget: If your supplement program does not contain L-citrulline to synergize the L-arginine, you will not receive the full benefit of Say Yes to NO.

A Blessed Event

Joanne and Terry were devastated to learn that their newborn daughter was suffering from a life-threatening respiratory disorder called persistent pulmonary hypertension of the newborn, or PPHN.

Their doctor told them that the cause of this very serious condition has yet to be determined, but the precipitating situation was the newborn's inability to begin breathing on her own. He explained that at birth, responding to the first few minutes of breathing air, the blood vessels in the lungs of a normal infant relax so that blood can flow through them and exchange carbon dioxide, a waste product, for oxygen. In their baby's case, her cardiovascular system could not make the adaptation, and the result was extremely high pulmonary blood pressure, which, if not addressed, could cause systemic damage, even death. When the couple asked what could be done for their baby, their physician broke into a smile.

"If it was even ten years ago, I wouldn't be smiling," he began, "but in 1997, two studies financed by the March of Dimes found that nitric oxide—a gas produced by the body to relax blood vessels—when inhaled by infants with PPHN lowered their blood pressure and greatly improved the newborns' condition. In addition, the nitric oxide method was noninvasive and made risky surgery unnecessary. I urge you to do it."

Since Terry associated nitric oxide with polluting car exhaust, he was a bit skeptical, but he and Joanne had total trust in their doctor, so they told him to go ahead.

The result seemed like a miracle to Joanne and Terry. Not only did their baby recover completely, but it is now four years later and she is in perfect health.

WEIGHING THE EVIDENCE

Though anecdotal stories are intriguing, as a scientist I know the shortcomings of case reports. Fortunately, we can now turn to a growing body of research confirming what the anecdotal accounts have suggested. If you have high blood pressure, elevated cholesterol levels, or atherosclerosis, L-arginine generated by L-citrulline can help restore the endothelium in your blood vessels, increase the body's production of NO, and improve your cardiovascular well-being.

Let's look at more of the research demonstrating the effectiveness of L-arginine in boosting NO levels and enhancing heart health:

Intravenous L-Arginine Testing

Some early research involved intravenous administration of L-arginine, in which the amino acid was delivered directly into the bloodstream, bypassing the need for absorption through the digestive system. Not only can intravenous dosing produce more rapid effects than if L-arginine is taken orally, but only a fraction of the oral dose is necessary to have a positive impact. Here are descriptions of two of these studies:

- In research at Keio University School of Medicine in Tokyo, five patients with high blood pressure (average readings of 155/95 mm Hg) were given IV doses of L-arginine. During administration of the amino acid, both systolic and diastolic blood pressure readings declined, achieving a mean decrease of 30 mm Hg and 22 mm Hg, respectively.

- Boston University's School of Medicine tested intravenous L-arginine generated from L-citrulline as a means to ameliorate cellular damage in a subject with a depressed cardiovascular profile endothelial function. Researchers found that the administration of either L-arginine or L-citrulline results in increased production of NO, which in turn relaxes the blood vessels, improves blood delivery to the organs, lowers blood pressure, and prevents unwanted blood clotting.

L-Arginine Nutraceuticals Testing

Infusions of L-arginine are fine for research studies, but they are impractical for day-to-day living. Other studies have examined whether L-arginine supplements can have an equally positive influence on cardiovascular health. Here are highlights from that research:

- In 1995, researchers at Sinai Hospital in Baltimore reported their study, in which forty-five healthy, elderly volunteers were given either an L-arginine supplement (17 grams per day) or placebo. After fourteen days, blood tests showed decreases in both total and LDL ("bad") cholesterol, without any changes in HDL cholesterol. There were no side effects noted with the L-arginine supplements.

- At Stanford University's Division of Cardiovascular Medicine, researchers set out to determine whether L-arginine supplementation could reduce blood platelet stickiness in individuals with high blood cholesterol levels. They placed patients on oral L-arginine supplements (8.4 grams a day) or placebo. After two weeks, platelet aggregation was modestly reduced in the people taking L-arginine—an effect that continued for another two weeks after the L-arginine supplementation had been stopped. The platelet activity returned to baseline levels eighteen weeks after the last supplements were taken. No side effects associated with L-arginine were reported. The researchers noted that these findings were similar to those in previous animal studies, which found that L-arginine restored NO activity while interfering with platelet aggregation.

NO Produces Incredible Results

"After three weeks on NO-boosting supplements, my blood pressure went from 163/94 to 124/80—with no blood pressure medication!"

Cathy, 55, Topeka

THE VERDICT IS IN

If you take L-arginine and L-citrulline supplements in combination with the antioxidants I recommend, you will begin to experience their positive effects in just weeks. If you have high blood pressure, for example, and the prescription antihypertensive medications you are taking have not lowered your levels to normal, L-arginine may reduce your blood pressure readings into the safe range by dilating your blood vessels.

Your doctor might be so impressed by the decline in your blood pressure that he may reduce your dose of prescription medications, or perhaps even eliminate them altogether. Any changes in your medication should be made only under your doctor's supervision.

SAY YES TO ANTIOXIDANTS

Antioxidants—whether they come from your diet or from supplements—can further step up NO production by deactivating or neutralizing dangerous free radicals, which are created during the process known as oxidative stress. By waging war on free radicals, antioxidants can restore the health of your NO-producing endothelial cells and guard against future deficits in NO production.

NO More Smoke and Mirrors

You cannot step into a health-food store these days without encountering stacks of hyped-up literature and a blizzard of colorful product labels that often make startling claims—many of them thoroughly unsubstantiated—about the health-enhancing properties of various pills and potions.

Though you should not give in to all the smoke and mirrors, some supplements—specifically those described in this chapter—are vital to your heart health. They can make an important difference in your well-being.

I have concentrated on only the important antioxidants—those with *proven* benefits for cardiovascular health and which are known to be safe in the doses I recommend. If you focus on incorporating just these antioxidants into your daily diet and supplement regimen, you can make some dramatic improvements in your health, now and in the future.

Are Antioxidants for Real?

In the past several years there have been a few studies reported in the popular press that seem to conclude that antioxidants are often of no benefit to cardiovascular health, and in some cases even harmful. The publicity has left many patients—and even some doctors—in doubt as to what to believe. If you are among those who have questions, rest assured that my recommended antioxidant levels in both supplement and food form will not be damaging to your health.

As an August 2004 article in the *Journal of the American Medical Association* pointed out, there have been decades of published studies showing the therapeutic benefits of antioxidants like vitamin E. Hundreds of careful experiments show clearly that antioxidants slow the progression of atherosclerosis. The article noted that the studies with negative results were not truly comparable to the existing body of knowledge, because the clinical trial methods differed in a number of important aspects, such as selection of subjects, stage of disease, end points, dosage, and source of the vitamin. Contradictory evidence from a few recent studies on isolated antioxidants cannot negate the benefits that have already been known for years. I would challenge the merits of these negative clinical trials before accepting any new dogma that antioxidants are not beneficial for the heart.

Even more important, within the context of nitric oxide enhancement there is one point that supersedes all others: the combination of L-arginine plus antioxidants is completely different in principle from antioxidants alone. Nitric oxide is produced from L-arginine, and the antioxidants act to stabilize and protect the nitric oxide as it is created, thereby further elevating the levels of nitric oxide. A large body of clinical reports shows that the combination of L-arginine plus antioxidants is of great benefit to humans. These tests are fundamentally different from the few that discount the benefits of antioxidants, which are tests of the effects produced by antioxidants alone.

So, are antioxidants for real? Clearly it is not really necessary to answer that question when talking about NO. The relevant question is "Is the combination of L-arginine and antioxidants for real?" The answer is an emphatic yes. Moreover, as I mentioned earlier, nitric oxide itself is the most potent antioxidant in the body, and no scientist would ever deny the fact that NO is the body's most important protector of heart health. My confidence in antioxidants has not been shaken by a few press reports, and neither should yours be.

Supplements or Diet or Both?

You would have to consume enormous quantities of foods rich in vitamins C and E to obtain adequate amounts of these nutraceuticals from your diet alone. For example, to reach 500 mg of vitamin C—the dosage I recommend—you would have to consume *five* 8-ounce glasses of orange juice. Even if you managed to do so, you would be flooding your body with sugar and calories.

Dr. Ignarro's Cardiovascular RDA

Most people are familiar with the RDAs, or Recommended Dietary Allowances. These guidelines were first issued in the 1940s by the Food and Nutrition Board of the National Academy of Science's National Research Council, and they have been revised periodically. When the RDAs were initially established, they were set at levels designed to prevent nutritional deficiencies, not to ensure optimal cardiovascular health.

In order to neutralize free radicals and protect your cardiovascular system from serious chronic diseases, I believe you need to take NO-boosting nutrients at levels higher than the RDAs. Nutraceuticals provide a safe and effective way of consuming optimal levels of these antioxidants, no matter how much or how little you are consuming in your diet.

Let's explore in depth the antioxidants that should be part of your own NO-supportive supplement program.

SAY YES TO VITAMIN C

Since two-time Nobel laureate Linus Pauling began heralding vitamin C for the prevention and treatment of just about everything that ails you—from the common cold to cancer—some Americans have become true believers in this vitamin, particularly at very high doses. Pauling insisted that by consuming 1 gram (1000 mg) of vitamin C a day, you could prevent the common cold. He claimed that once you already had a cold, several grams a day could cure it.

Of course, you can get vitamin C in your diet by eating lots of oranges and other citrus fruit, strawberries, melons, tomatoes, brussels sprouts, cauliflower, broccoli, and spinach—but at the levels I recommend, you will probably need to take a supplement as well. I am convinced that you need more vitamin C than the RDA suggests to enjoy the full cardiovascular benefits of this very important antioxidant.

The Story of Vitamin C

Vitamin C actually came to prominence in the early 1930s when a Hungarian researcher, Albert Szent-Gyorgyi, first isolated the vitamin. He was awarded the Nobel Prize in 1937 for his discovery. Vitamin C was identified as the substance in fruits and vegetables capable of preventing and curing scurvy, a disease that for centuries had been responsible for the deaths of thousands of sailors who subsisted for months on diets without vitamin C–rich fruits and vegetables. Szent-Gyorgyi used the term *ascorbic acid* to describe this newly identified substance.

Today, we know that vitamin C is a water-soluble vitamin. In other words, it dissolves in water. Your body absorbs it through the gastrointestinal tract, and excess amounts are excreted in the urine rather than stored in the body.

Vitamin C as a Potent Anti-Cancer Weapon

Scientists at the National Cancer Institute conducted a study involving 10,000 men and women, analyzing their dietary histories and then monitoring them for the following nineteen years. In an article published in the *American Journal of Epidemiology* in 1997, those individuals with the highest intakes of vitamin C had a 34 percent lower risk of developing lung cancer than those who consumed the least amount of vitamin C.

What Vitamin C Can Do for Your Health

The many functions of vitamin C in the body include:

- Playing a role in the formation of collagen—an important protein in the body's connective tissue.
- Stimulating the healing of wounds.
- Facilitating the absorption of iron from the intestinal tract, thus reducing the risk of iron-deficiency anemia.
- Maintaining a healthy immune system by playing a critical role in the production of various antibodies that can resist bacteria and viruses.

- Guarding the body against free radicals and the potentially devastating injuries they cause, including damage to the cardiovascular system.

- Acting as a shield that protects health-enhancing nitric oxide.

The human body does not manufacture vitamin C. For that reason, your diet and your use of supplements become even more important in ensuring that you consume sufficient amounts of this nutrient.

Vitamin C: Essential to Cardiovascular Health

At the UCLA School of Public Health, investigators looked at the relationship between vitamin C consumption and mortality in more than 11,300 adults over a period of ten years. In their study published in *Epidemiology* in 1992, the individuals who consumed the most vitamin C (more than 50 mg per day) were more likely to remain free of disease than those with a lower intake. The higher-consumption group not only had a lower overall death rate, but also a lower risk of death from both heart disease and cancer.

Vitamin C: Dr. Ignarro's Cardiovascular RDA

Medical science has convinced me of the importance of vitamin C to overall cardiovascular health—in doses greater than the RDA's recommendation of 60 mg a day for adults. There is plenty of evidence to show that a higher intake can improve endothelial function, lower blood pressure readings, and reduce your risk of heart disease. Yes, it is very important to include plenty of vitamin C–rich foods in your diet, but I suggest you take a daily vitamin C supplement as well.

Vitamin C: Dr. Ignarro's Cardiovascular RDA	500 mg of vitamin C supplement daily

At a daily dosage of 500 mg, your intake is at a safe level, both in the short term and after taking the vitamin for months, even years.

Are Natural Vitamins More Effective Than Synthetic Ones?

Browse through the vitamin section of a health-food store, and you will see natural and synthetic forms of many products. You might find yourself attracted to the "natural" pills and capsules, convinced that "natural is better." Natural products—or nutraceuticals—are more expensive. Since they are extracted from food—not produced in a laboratory like synthetic products—you might believe the argument that they are a healthier option.

That is not true. Despite the hyperbole associated with natural vitamins, they have exactly the same chemical structure as the synthetic products. The word "natural" may be comforting, but they perform no differently in the body than the synthetic versions.

The bottom line is that synthetic vitamins are the real thing. Chemically, they are identical to natural vitamins. They provide exactly the same benefits. Vitamin C is vitamin C, whether it is extracted from an orange or a grapefruit or synthesized in a manufacturing plant.

In much the same way, a vitamin C product that is "derived from rose hips" offers no special advantages. Yes, rose hips, the seed pods or the "hip" of the rose, are an excellent source of vitamin C, but the quality of the rose hips vitamin is no better than what you would find in a synthetic product. In fact, it is not unusual for some "rose hip vitamins" to be primarily synthetic.

Vitamin C: Weighing the Evidence

Here is just a sampling of some of the impressive research demonstrating the benefits of vitamin C.

- At the University of Tennessee, in a study published in the journal *Circulation* in 1995, researchers evaluated the effects of vitamin C on more than 11,000 patients. They found that men and women over age fifty-five who consumed high levels of vitamin C experienced less thickening of their carotid arteries, compared to individuals who consumed lower amounts. The conclusion of the investigators: Vitamin C appears to protect against atherosclerotic disease.
- Researchers at the University of Kuopio in Finland looked at the effects of antioxidants on the blood pres-

sure of more than 700 men participating in the Kuo-pio Ischaemic Heart Disease Risk Factor Study. In the *American Journal of Clinical Nutrition* in 1988 they reported that both systolic and diastolic blood pressure readings were an average of about 5 percent lower in the men with the highest blood levels of vitamin C (ascorbic acid), compared to the subjects with the lowest blood levels. Reported in the *Journal of the American Medical Association* in 1997, a study conducted at the University of Maryland School of Medicine examined the effects of a high dose of vitamin C on the functioning of the endothelium. Healthy volunteers were given either (a) a single high-fat meal consisting of 50 grams of fat, (b) a low-fat meal with 0 grams of fat, or (c) a high-fat (50 gram) meal after taking 1000 mg of vitamin C and 800 IU of vitamin E. In the high-fat meal group without the antioxidants, measurements with ultrasound scans showed that the enormous fat intake interfered with the normal dilation of their arteries and their blood flow, known as the "endothelium-dependent artery vasodilation" for up to four hours. The group eating the same fat-laden meal but taking vitamins did not experience any such negative effects. These individuals had normal dilation and normal blood flow to the heart. As the researchers concluded, "a single high-fat meal reduced endothelial function for up to four hours" in healthy people with normal cholesterol levels, "this decrease is blocked by pretreatment with antioxidant vitamins C and E."

SAY YES TO VITAMIN E

Vitamin E is another potent antioxidant crucial to maximizing the levels of NO in your body and protecting your cardiovascular health. Unlike vitamin C, it is a fat-soluble vitamin—that is, it dissolves only in liquid fats and not in water—and can be stored in the body once it is absorbed through the membranes of the intestines. Vitamin E's history dates back to 1922, when researchers Herbert Evans and Katherine Bishop at the University of California, Berkeley, discovered a substance capable of influencing the reproductive ability of laboratory animals but the effect of which on humans was a mystery. Some investigators referred to it as "Factor X."

Researchers have discussed and debated the functions of vitamin E ever since. For a time, Factor X was called "a vitamin in search of a disease," largely because there was no definitive evidence that a deficiency of vitamin E could trigger any particular illness or symptoms in humans. The research has continued and the evidence has accumulated. Today, vitamin E's importance to human health is much clearer, although admittedly not absolute.

What Vitamin E Can Do for Your Health

We now know that vitamin E is actually a group of compounds—the tocopherols and tocotrienols. Alpha-tocopherol, the most biologically active form of the ·vitamin, is widely found in small amounts in foods, particularly vegetable oils—including corn, soybean, and safflower—wheat germ, and nuts. I recommend that you incorporate alpha-tocopherol into your personal antioxidant program. Vitamin E may well play an important role in interfering with inflammatory processes within your body, which are known to exacerbate cardiovascular disease. Vitamin E also appears to impede the formation of LDL cholesterol.

Vitamin E Reduces Heart Attacks!

At Cambridge University in the United Kingdom, researchers in the Cambridge Heart Antioxidant Study (CHAOS) looked at the effects of vitamin E on 2,002 individuals with confirmed heart disease. Slightly more than half the subjects were given alpha-tocopherol capsules (some at a dose of 800 IU a day, others at 400 IU) for a median of 510 days; the remainder were placed on placebo capsules. In findings published in the journal *Lancet* in 1996, the investigators reported that the group taking the active vitamin experienced a dramatic 77 percent reduced risk of nonfatal heart attacks, compared to those receiving a placebo. The benefits of the vitamin were seen within six and a half months after the volunteers began taking the supplements.

Vitamin E: Dr. Ignarro's Cardiovascular RDA

The government RDA for Vitamin E is only 12 IU for adult women and 15 IU for adult men. Yet to optimize its benefits, I recommend that you take a much higher but still safe dose. Most studies indicate that therapeutic doses of vitamin E can range as high as 1000 IU, and often higher, without the risk of side effects.

Vitamin E: Dr. Ignarro's Cardiovascular RDA	200 IU of vitamin E supplement daily

Vitamin E (alpha-tocopherol) can be purchased in capsule form.

Caution: A Risk Factor

Because vitamin E has mild blood-thinning properties, talk to your doctor, especially if you are already taking an anticoagulant or blood thinner such as Coumadin or aspirin, often prescribed to counteract the clotting mechanism in order to reduce your risk of a heart attack or stroke. Your physician might recommend that you refrain from using vitamin E supplements to avoid magnifying the blood-thinning properties of the drugs your doctor has already prescribed.

Vitamin E: Weighing the Evidence

Many studies now confirm that vitamin E can undermine oxidative stress within the body. As it does, it neutralizes free radicals before they can cause cardiovascular or other serious diseases. Here is just some of the most persuasive evidence:

- The well-known Nurses' Health Study by Harvard researchers followed 87,245 female nurses (ages thirty-four to fifty-nine) for up to eight years. All of these women had been free of diagnosed cardiovascular disease when the study began. The investigators evaluated those women who consumed the greatest amount of vitamin E in their diet during this time, and compared them to women who had the lowest intake of the vitamin. In an article published in the *New England Journal of Medicine* in 1993, they concluded that the women with the highest vitamin E intake had a 34 percent lower risk of developing major coronary disease than those with the lowest intake. In women who took vitamin E supplements (100 IU or more) per day for over two years, their risk declined 41 percent.

- Data from a parallel study at Harvard, the Health Professionals Study, were published in the same journal in 1993. It examined nearly 40,000 male health professionals (ages forty to seventy-five), who had been free of diagnosed coronary heart disease when the study began. After four years of follow-up, those men whose intake of vitamin E was more than 60 IU per day had a 36 percent lower risk of developing coronary disease than those whose intake was less than 7.5 IU per day. Among the men who took daily vitamin E supplements of 100 IU per day for at least two years, their likelihood of having coronary disease was 37 percent lower than those who did not take supplements.

- At the University of Texas Southwestern Medical Center, researchers gave twenty-one healthy individuals supplements of vitamin E (1,200 IU per day), and monitored their levels of oxidized LDL cholesterol. After eight weeks of taking vitamin E supplements, the twenty-one subjects experienced significant declines in the propensity of their LDL cholesterol to become oxidized by free radicals. In the *Journal of Clinical Investigation* in 1996, the Texas scientists also reported a significant decline in the quantity of free radicals discharged by monocytes, a type of white blood cell that can adhere to the endothelial wall.

"Factor X," now known as vitamin E, has become a boon to medical science in general—and cardiovascular health in particular.

SAY YES TO FOLIC ACID

Folic acid is a B vitamin and is an extremely important ingredient of my antioxidant package, but not because it necessarily has powerful antioxidant properties in its own right. Folic acid is a "co-factor." It must be present in order for certain enzymes to perform their crucial functions in the body, including some that decrease the activity of free radicals. If you can interfere with oxidative stress, you can stabilize the NO in your body. At the same time, folic acid helps sustain the activity of NO synthase, which maintains NO production at full throttle.

The Story of Folic Acid

In the 1920s, a baffling cluster of deaths occurred among pregnant women in Bombay, India. These young women were found to have a form of anemia, and their condition was labeled "pregnancy anemia." Although there were many unanswered questions about this wave of illness, its victims tended to be poorly nourished, living on a diet of mostly bread and polished rice. Even so, they did not seem to have deficiencies in iron or other nutrients typically associated with anemia.

Desperate for a treatment, some doctors began giving extracts of yeast and liver to their pregnant, anemic patients. To their surprise, these women returned to good health. It took more than another decade to gain a better understanding of what had taken place.

Scientists pinpointed an unidentified vitamin, present in these foods, as a key in the scenario involving the pregnant women. In the 1940s, researchers were able to manufacture an extract of the vitamin from the leaves of spinach. They named it "folic acid" from the Latin *folium,* meaning *leaf.* A healthy intake of folic acid is important for everyone, not just pregnant women, including those interested in nurturing their cardiovascular health.

What Folic Acid Can Do for Your Health

Another important function of folic acid is that it can lower your blood levels of homocysteine, an amino acid that is a risk factor for cardiovascular disease. Even though a Harvard pathologist, Kilmer McCully, first proposed an association between severe atherosclerosis and high homocysteine levels in 1969, his hypothesis gained little support until the 1990s, when research began confirming what McCully had seen decades earlier. A solid body of research now shows that in individuals with high blood levels of homocysteine, the risk of heart attacks is much higher than in people with low levels. Homocysteine appears to injure the endothelial cells responsible for the body's production of NO.

The good news is that folic acid (B_9), along with B_6 and B_{12}, can reduce the levels of homocysteine in the bloodstream. Folic acid is certainly available in foods, including leafy green vegetables, whole grains, oranges, egg yolks, legumes, liver, nuts, fortified breakfast cereals, breads, and pasta. But you can also consume it in supplement form, which is a more reliable way of ensuring that you receive the proper amount of folic acid required by your body as an antioxidant and NO-booster.

Folic Acid: A Key to Endothelial Wellness

Researchers at the Harvard School of Public Health wrote a review article that described a series of studies examining the ability of an individual's diet to modify the functioning of the endothelium. Their article, published in the *American Journal of Clinical Nutrition* in 2001, concluded that the "overall results of these studies suggest that folic acid supplementation has a beneficial effect on endothelial function . . . in healthy subjects or patients with elevated homocysteine." The scientists wrote that this benefit "is probably explained largely by the homocysteine-lowering effect of folic acid," although they also noted that this B vitamin is found to have some antioxidant properties in laboratory research and "may directly improve nitric-oxide production by enhancing enzymatic activity of nitric-oxide synthase."

Optimal Level of Folic Acid

With folic acid's ability to slash homocysteine levels, what level of this important B vitamin is optimal? That was the question addressed by British researchers in a study published in the *Archives of Internal Medicine* in 2001. In this clinical trial, 151 adults with heart disease were placed on one of five doses of folic acid (200, 400, 800, or 1,000 mcg) or a placebo daily for three months. The data showed that every dose of folic acid reduced the levels of homocysteine in the blood—and the higher the homocysteine levels, the greater the decline. The maximum decreases in homocysteine occurred with the daily dose of 800 mcg. In the people taking the 800 mcg dose, homocysteine levels fell 23 percent, compared to the placebo group. The researchers concluded that a dosage of 800 mcg of folic acid per day appears necessary to achieve the maximum decrease in homocysteine levels.

Folic Acid: Dr. Ignarro's Cardiovascular RDA

The federal RDA of folic acid was recently increased from 180 to 400 mcg. My recommendation is to take a daily supplement of 400 to 800 mcg of folic acid, which is the level found to produce maximum benefits in the British study cited above. At this level, folic acid is a safe vitamin. Even at higher doses, there is no research indicating any adverse effects.

Folic Acid (Vitamin B9): Dr. Ignarro's Cardiovascular RDA	400 to 800 mcg of folic acid supplement daily

Folic Acid: Weighing the Evidence

Here are the findings of some amazing folic acid studies:

- In an article published in the *Journal of the American Medical Association* in 1997, researchers at nineteen cen-

ters throughout Europe participating in the European
Concerted Action Project, studied 750 people with
atherosclerotic vascular disease along with 800 control
subjects without the disease. They found that individuals with high blood levels of homocysteine had a
significantly increased risk of heart disease. When patients took supplements that contained folic acid, vitamin B_6, and vitamin B_{12}, their risk of heart disease
plummeted 62 percent.

- At the University of California, San Diego, researchers
  conducted a trial involving 553 patients who had already undergone a successful angioplasty to open arterial blockages. The investigators wanted to determine
  whether vitamin therapy that included folic acid could
  lower their levels of homocysteine in the blood and
  reduce the risk of restenosis, a renarrowing of the arteries at the same location where the angioplasty treatment occurred. Participants were randomly assigned
  to receive either a combination of folic acid (1 mg per
  day), vitamins B_6 (10 mg per day), and B_{12} (400 mcg
  per day), or a placebo for six months. In the *Journal of
  the American Medical Association* in 2002, the researchers
  reported that after a mean eleven months of follow-
  up, those individuals receiving the vitamin therapy had
  a significantly lower need for a repeat angioplasty as
  well as a reduced overall incidence of heart attacks and
  death—even though they had been taken off the vitamin therapy for the last several months of evaluation.
  The patients receiving placebo had a 37.6 percent
  restenosis rate, compared to 19.6 percent among those
  taking the B vitamins.

SAY YES TO ALPHA LIPOIC ACID

Most people are familiar with alpha lipoic acid (ALA) as an ingredient in skin care products, even though we are learning that it is a potent scavenger that can neutralize many types of free radicals when ingested. ALA appears to be both a water- and a fat-soluble substance, and because of its fat-soluble properties, it resides in cell membranes and can prevent those membranes from being destroyed by free radical activity. ALA can also enter the water-based portions of the cells, where it can provide further protection.

The Story of Alpha Lipoic Acid

The antioxidant function of alpha lipoic acid was first investigated in the late thirties. By the early forties, research studies were able to prove that the antioxidant ALA fought free radicals.

By 1951, researchers had learned that ALA is naturally found in the cells of the body that generate energy. When alpha lipoic acid production is boosted, it enters those cells and protects its molecules from being plundered by unstable free radicals trying to replace their missing molecules and return to stability.

What ALA Can Do for Your Health

Following are the proven benefits of ALA:

- ALA can trigger chemical reactions in the body that increase or recycle the levels of other key antioxidants, including vitamins C and E.

- It can increase the amount of nitric oxide, as well as improve the stability and duration of the action of NO.

- It can facilitate glucose metabolism and is often recommended for people with diabetes.

- In animal studies, ALA has decreased blood pressure readings, protected the brain from stroke-related injuries, and improved the functioning of the vascular system.

Alpha Lipoic Acid: Dr. Ignarro's Cardiovascular RDA

Alpha Lipoic Acid (ALA): Dr. Ignarro's Cardiovascular RDA	10 mg of alpha lipoic acid supplement daily

Alpha Lipoic Acid: Weighing the Evidence

Here are just two of the recent studies evaluating the effects of alpha lipoic acid in the vascular system:

- In a particularly impressive animal study, reported in *Brain Research* in 1996, researchers in India and the U.S. induced a stroke in laboratory rats by manipulating the carotid artery leading to the brain. When they restored the blood flow, there was a surge in oxygen radicals, and 78 percent of the animals died after twenty-four hours. Then the experiment was performed again, but this time the rats were given alpha lipoic acid just before the blood flow was reestablished. Twenty-four hours later, the death rate had fallen to 26 percent, indicating that this antioxidant may have protected the animal brains against injury as the blood flow resumed.

- Canadian researchers divided hypertensive rats into groups, with one of them receiving a diet supplemented with alpha lipoic acid, while another was fed a normal diet without ALA. After nine weeks, systolic blood pressure readings were significantly lower in the group given the antioxidant supplementation. These systolic measurements decreased from a mean of 180 mm Hg to 140 mm Hg in the ALA group, while the untreated animals experienced an *increase* in pressure from 180 to 195 mm Hg. There were also indications of structural improvements in the vascular system with ALA, including reductions in vascular damage and decreased evidence of atherosclerosis.

GETTING THE MOST FROM SAY YES TO NO SUPPLEMENTS

There are many other antioxidants that I have not included here—from beta-carotene and pycnogenol to selenium and garlic. After careful consideration and evaluation, I decided that by concentrating on the select group of amino acids and antioxidants offering the most potent cardiovascular aid, you will achieve maximum benefits through the synergy of taking them together. With the primary goal of preserving and maximizing the efficacy of nitric oxide, these are the four antioxidants you should be taking.

Summary of NO Supplements

L-arginine	4–6 g (4000–6000 mg) per day
L-citrulline	200–1000 mg per day
Vitamin C	500 mg per day
Vitamin E (alpha-tocopherol)	200 IU per day
Folic acid (Vitamin B₉)	400–800 mcg per day
Alpha lipoic acid	10 mg per day

These supplements can be taken with or without food. There is no evidence that any of their components will cause gastric irritation if you take them on an empty stomach. Many people tell me that if they take the supplements at the same time every day—perhaps before or after breakfast or lunch—they are more likely to remember to use them daily as they become part of a routine. Whenever you decide to take the supplements, be sure that you take all of them, in the correct dosages, in order to activate the benefits of **Say Yes to NO.**

NO: Easy on the Heart, Easy on the Tummy

Maureen, a vivacious New York personal trainer in her mid-fifties, is devoted to fitness. She practices heart-healthy nutrition and works out regularly. For years, Maureen had been trying to take vitamin supplements, but, after a couple of weeks, they upset her stomach so badly, she had to discontinue them. Then she discovered NO-boosting supplements in powder form. "After a couple of

> months, I've had absolutely no digestive problems,
> I sleep like a baby, and have twice the energy I did a year
> ago. And I'm protecting my cardiovascular health at the
> same time!"

SHOPPING FOR SUPPLEMENTS

If you are planning to take the NO-boosting nutraceuticals in pill form, you can do all your shopping without leaving your house—because all the sources I recommend have Web sites from which you can order. Shopping online makes it much easier to assemble your supplements one by one, because you will never have to drive all over town, trudging from store to store, in order to find the different products you need.

When it comes to purchasing supplements on the Internet, I am a great admirer of several currently existing sites, for example: Life Extension (www.LifeExtension.com); their products are of the highest quality while their prices are among the most reasonable around. I am also partial to the GNC stores (www.GNC.com), Savon (www.Savon.com), and of course Drugstore.com (www.Drugstore.com).

Shopping for L-arginine

Recommended dosage: 4–6 g (4000–6000 mg) daily
L-arginine is available in capsule form from GNC, Savon, Life Extension, and Drugstore.com.

Shopping for L-citrulline

Recommended dosage: 200–1000 mg daily

Until recently, it was virtually impossible to find L-citrulline as a stand-alone dietary supplement, but that is changing. If you do a search on the Internet by asking "where can I purchase pure L-citrulline?" you will be directed to several pill or powder alternatives.

Shopping for Vitamin C

Recommended dosage: 500 mg daily

Vitamin C is available anywhere and everywhere: Life Extension, GNC, Savon, Drugstore.com, and many other sites.

Shopping for Vitamin E (alpha-tocopherol)

Recommended dosage: 200 IU daily

Like vitamin C, vitamin E is available anywhere and everywhere: Life Extension, GNC, Savon, Drugstore.com, and many other sites.

Shopping for Folic Acid

Recommended dosage: 400–800 mcg daily

Like Vitamins C and E, folic acid can found anywhere and everywhere: Life Extension, GNC, Savon, Drugstore.com, and many other sites.

Shopping for Alpha Lipoic Acid

Recommended dosage: 10 mg daily

I suggest purchasing alpha lipoic acid from Life Extension, GNC, Savon, or Drugstore.com.

A Powdered Alternative

Until recently the only way to take all of my recommended supplements was to obtain nutrients separately and spend a great deal of time and effort taking pills. I have recently designed an alternative that delivers the appropriate amounts of my select group of nutrients in the form of powder that is dissolved in water and then drunk. This powdered supplement, called Niteworks, is the only product I am aware of on the market with the proper amounts of L-arginine and L-citrulline, thereby enabling the full synergistic effects of the **Say Yes to NO** program.

No matter in what form you take the **Say Yes to NO** supplements, just do it. And be sure you take the amino acids and antioxidants together, because the synergy will stimulate your NO production even more.

Your body will notice the difference in a matter of weeks.

It's Working for Her

Dear Dr. Ignarro,

I've noticed several improvements in my overall health since being on your program for the past three months. Emotionally, I have a greater sense of well-being, and I don't seem to be as anxious about minor annoyances. On the physical side, I have better stamina, feel fewer muscle aches after hard work, and my neck and shoulder pains have gone away! These pains had plagued me my whole adult life. I have also had fewer bouts with allergies during the last two months. In the past, allergies and sinusitis have been extremely debilitating.

The most significant change is that I'm getting better sleep, which has been a major problem for me for years. I can't say with absolute certainty that your program has caused all these changes, but I doubt it is pure coincidence.

Sincerely,
Sally
Butte, Montana, USA

THE HEART OF THE MATTER

Before we move on, let's review what you learned in this chapter.

The first part of the chapter discussed L–arginine and L–citrulline and how they contribute to the production of NO:

- Scientists have discovered that the body can manufacture some L-arginine with the help of that other NO-boosting amino acid, L-citrulline, which is formed inside the cells of the body where it is converted to nitric oxide.

- The body can convert L-citrulline back to L-arginine and in the process prolong NO's brief life.

- The optimal dose for L-arginine supplements is 4 to 6 grams (4000 to 6000 mg) per day.

- The optimal dose for L-citrulline supplements is 200 to 1,000 mg per day.

The second part of the chapter discussed how antioxidants can protect against free radicals:

- Antioxidants can facilitate the body's production of nitric oxide by neutralizing oxygen radicals and restoring the health of NO-manufacturing endothelial cells.

- Generous amounts of vitamin C can improve endothelial function and enhance cardiovascular health. Although vitamin C is present in many foods, you will need more than the government's RDA to reap the benefits of this antioxidant, and thus supplementation is recommended.

- Folic acid is a "co-factor" that sustains the activity of the enzyme NO synthase, which promotes the body's manufacturing of nitric oxide and helps reduce the risk of heart attack.

- Alpha lipoic acid is present in cell membranes, minimizing the activity of oxygen radicals.

- When shopping for vitamins, keep in mind that there is no chemical difference between synthetic and "natural" supplements. The benefits they provide are identical.

- Antioxidants should be taken together with L-argi-nine and L-citrulline to maximize NO production. The synergy between these three elements of the **Say Yes to NO** supplement program is required to generate optimal health benefits.

7

SAY YES TO NO-BOOSTING NUTRITION

I take my NO-boosting supplements every single evening, whether I am at home or flying to Europe for a speaking engagement. Important as these nutraceuticals are, I know they can increase my nitric oxide production even more when they are synergized with NO-friendly functional foods. After you read this chapter, you will want to organize your meals around these foods, too.

The foundation for NO-boosting nutrition is similar to that for NO-boosting supplements. In Chapter 6, I discussed the importance of supplements for antioxidants like vitamins C and E, and for amino acids like L-arginine and L-citrulline, which all work to support either the direct or indirect action of nitric oxide. It is important to understand that all these essential fuels for the body are also available in a wide variety of foods.

In many cases even the most dedicated person cannot consume large enough quantities of these functional foods to meet the body's total NO requirement—hence the need for supplements. However, it is wise to provide as much of these critical nutrients as possible through your food intake. A major goal of the **Say Yes to NO** program is to show you that your body performs best when you feed it the nutrients it requires through the synergistic combination of supplements and the food you choose to eat.

In this chapter I will describe some important guidelines for NO-friendly meals—certainly not a rigid, restrictive diet plan, but a general approach to healthy, NO-rich eating.

NO-FRIENDLY FOODS

The good news is that there is a wide variety of foods to choose from that can enhance your NO production and overall health. Before launching into detailed discussion of many of the key factors you must understand about NO-friendly nutrition, I want to lay out for you a fairly comprehensive list of the different foods you can choose in the **Say Yes to NO**-boosting nutrition program. But be aware, this list is not completely exhaustive, so if there is a food you like that is not on the list, I urge you to check into its nutritional properties. You may find that it can support your health as well as some of the foods on the list.

Foods Rich in Antioxidants

Artichokes (cooked)

Avocado

Bananas

Black beans (dried)

Black plums

Blackberries

Blueberries (cultivated or
    wild)

Bran cereal

Broccoli

Brussels sprouts

Cantaloupe

Carrots

Celery

Chicken breast

Corn

Crab

Cranberries

Dark chocolate
Fish oil
Flaxseed
Gala apples
Garbanzo beans
Garlic
Grains
Granny Smith apples
Grapefruit
Grapes/Grape juice
Lettuce
Liver
Mangos
Nuts
Oranges
Oysters
Papaya
Peanut butter
Pecans
Pinto beans

Plums
Pomegranate juice
Prunes
Raspberries
Red delicious apples
Red kidney beans
Red meat (in moderation!)
Red wine (in moderation!)
Russet potatoes (cooked)
Salmon
Seeds
Small red beans (dried)
Soybeans
Spinach
Strawberries
Sweet cherries
Sweet potatoes
Tea (black and green)
Tomatoes
Wheat germ

Foods Rich in L-Arginine and L-Citrulline

Almonds
Dark chocolate
Garbanzo beans
Melons
Peanuts
Red meat (in moderation!)
Salmon
Soy
Walnuts

Foods Rich in Proteins

Almonds
Cod
Eggs
Hazelnuts
Lobster
Peanuts
Salmon
Shrimp
Snapper
Soybeans
Swordfish
Tuna
Walnuts

Foods Rich in Omega-3 Fatty Acids*

Anchovy
Canola oil
Cod liver oil
Flaxseed oil
Halibut
Herring
Mackerel
Pumpkin seeds
Salmon

*Omega-3 fatty acids improve cholesterol, reduce heart attack and stroke, and protect against fatal cardiac arrhythmia (irregular heartbeat).

Sardines
Swordfish
Tuna
Walnuts

Heart-Healthy Fats

Canola oil
Corn oil
Olive oil (pure and virgin)
Safflower oil
Sesame oil (light and dark)
Vegetable oil

Remember, these lists may be long, but they are not exhaustive. Use your common sense, and do not be afraid to do additional research into the particular nutritional qualities of any foods you are interested in. I find the Internet to be a wealth of information for this purpose, although you must be careful to turn to reliable sources of scientific knowledge.

SAY NO TO SATURATED FATS, TRANS FATS, AND DIETARY CHOLESTEROL

You have probably heard the term "saturated fat" used quite a bit, and most likely you have come to realize that it is unhealthy for you. Excess intake of saturated fats can produce a wide range of health problems, including an inability to produce sufficient quantities of nitric oxide.

Saturated Fat Saturated fats tend to harden at room temperature; lard is an easily recognizable example. The body processes saturated fats differently from monounsaturates and polyunsaturates. Excess intake of saturated fats creates an elevated level of LDL ("bad") cholesterol. By now you are familiar with the threat to cardiovascular health posed by high LDL cholesterol. It can contribute to the accumulation of fatty deposits and plaque on the arterial walls, which leads to damage to the endothelium, impairing your body's ability to make NO.

If your diet consists of a lot of animal products—particularly such fatty meats as beef, pork, lamb, veal, and poultry skin, and such dairy products as whole milk, cheese, and ice cream—you are probably relying too heavily on saturated fats, which can ravage your arteries and create something of a cardiovascular time bomb, just waiting to be detonated.

Trans Fats Trans fats, which raise LDL to dangerous levels, are the results of hydrogenation—a manufactured food process in which hydrogen is added to vegetable oil to lengthen shelf life. The following foods are high in trans fats, so be sure to avoid them, regardless of how good you might think they taste: packaged cakes, cookies, crackers, pastry; bread, butter and margarine; such snack foods as potato chips, taco chips, and popcorn; fried potatoes, and commercial salad dressings.

Dietary Cholesterol It has been pointed out that foods that contribute to elevated LDL cholesterol are usually high in saturated fat. Steer clear of or rarely eat organ meats like liver; processed meats like hot dogs and salami; fatty red meats like rib steak; egg yolks, cream cheese, rich cheeses like cheddar and triple crèmes, full-fat dairy products, and ice cream.

You cannot load your diet with saturated fats, trans fats, and

LDL cholesterol and expect to maximize your NO production. You would be working against it.

The Facts about Fat

I recommend that you cut back on the high-fat meats and the dairy products for the sake of your NO levels and the health of your heart. The same holds for certain plant oils—such "tropical" oils as palm oil, palm kernel oil, coconut oil—which are high in saturated fats.

You do not need to "de-fat" your diet completely, but you should take steps to reduce the saturated fats, trans fats, and dietary cholesterol you eat. With moderate dietary changes, you can make major improvements in your NO levels and the overall well-being of your heart.

If you are eating red meat more than occasionally, I think you should modify your carnivorous habits. Reduce the number of servings and the size of your portions. Choose leaner cuts and trim away all visible fat before cooking. Turn more often to chicken and fish, which have less saturated fat than beef. When selecting chicken, choose white meat, be sure the skin is removed, and bake, broil or roast it.

Say Yes to Heart-Healthy Fats

Keep in mind that saturated fats are the cause of most fat-related cardiovascular problems, including high cholesterol. Other types of fat—monounsaturated fats in olive oil and canola oil, for example, and polyunsaturated fats in corn oil, sunflower oil, and safflower oil—are fats with high caloric counts. Still, they are better for you than saturated fat. In fact, growing scientific evidence shows that monounsaturates and polyunsaturates in moderation may actually maintain or even increase your HDL ("good") cholesterol levels while reducing the LDL.

Following is a list of heart-healthy fats recommended by the American Heart Association:

- *Canola oil*: It has approximately 60 percent less saturated fats than any other oil.

- *Corn oil*: Excellent for cooking because it can tolerate high temperatures without smoking.

- *Safflower oil*: Good for salads because it will not solidify in the refrigerator.

- *Light and dark sesame oil*: The dark version, made from toasted sesame seeds, is too intense to use for cooking and is considered a flavoring element; the light, made from untoasted sesame seeds, is extremely good for cooking.

- *Vegetable oil*: Most vegetable oils are made from soybeans, making them especially healthy—high in polyunsaturated and monounsaturated fat but low in saturated fat.

And last but not least . . .

- *Pure and virgin olive oil*: Entirely monounsaturated. Pure olive oil is heated when it is processed, while virgin is "cold pressed" and has a milder flavor.

  Since olive oil seems to be of special value to your cardiovascular system, strongly consider it when you are opting for "good" fats in your diet.

Can Extra Virgin Olive Oil Reduce Blood Pressure?

At the University of Naples in Italy, researchers evaluated the blood pressure-lowering effects of extra virgin olive oil, compared to sunflower oil, in hypertensive patients over a six-month period. As the scientists reported in the *Archives of Internal Medicine* in 2000, diets enriched with olive oil produced blood pressure readings significantly lower than those in the sunflower-oil group. Just as impressively, those taking olive oil were able to reduce their dosage of antihypertensive prescription medications by 48 percent, compared to 4 percent when sunflower oil was consumed.

Liquid Gold

If you look at the medical history books, you will find that olive oil was praised by Greek physician Hippocrates as "the great therapeutic" more than 2,000 years ago, while Greek poet Homer referred to it as "liquid gold." Since olive oil is so rich in flavor, you do not have to use much of it as a dressing on your salad or as an addition to sauces or marinades.

Kids at Risk

Now that there is a virtual epidemic of juvenile obesity and type II diabetes in America, could early onset hypertension be far behind? Dr. Bonita Falkner of Philadelphia's Thomas Jefferson University is the chairman of a government committee setting new guidelines for the treatment of high blood pressure in children. She says that as many as 3 percent of American children had high blood pressure with 10 percent more considered prehypertensive—and that diet and exercise are the first lines of defense.

If your child is hypertensive, you might want to discuss my **Say Yes to NO** regimen with his pediatrician. The nutrition is heart-healthy, the exercise can initially be moderate, and the supplements seem to behave in children as in adults—lowering blood pressure and keeping it down.

DON'T FORGET YOUR FIBER

Science has long known that a high-fiber diet is beneficial to the digestive system, even helping to prevent colon cancer. Now one study after another has suggested that a high intake of dietary fiber has been associated with lower rates of coronary artery disease.

As you reduce the portion sizes of foods high in saturated fat, substitute such fiber-rich foods as vegetables, fruit, whole-grain breads and cereals, beans, and brown rice. Most fiber passes through the body undigested in the stomach or intestines and is resistant to the activity of enzymes in the digestive tract. Fiber's job is to make sure everything in the body is moving smoothly before it exits the scene. Many fiber-rich foods like beans and oat bran contain mostly soluble fiber, which dissolves in water. Others are high in insoluble fiber—roughage that does not dissolve in water—such as grains, fruits, and vegetables.

Fiber and NO

Studies have suggested that soluble fiber can perform such antioxidant tasks as lowering blood pressure and LDL cholesterol levels and increasing HDL cholesterol—thereby protecting the endothelial cells where nitric oxide is manufactured. We are now coming to believe that fiber works through substances called *phytonutrients,* which seem to have the antioxidant advantage when it comes to guarding NO.

What are Phytonutrients?

Phytonutrients are nutrients found largely in the skins of many fruits and vegetables, where they produce the color, scent, and flavor. They are also contained, to a lesser extent, in grains and seeds. Phytonutrients are not vitamins; they are biologically active components of pigments whose full benefits are still being uncovered by researchers. Many of the foods recommended in **Say Yes to NO**–boosting nutrition contain large quantities of phytonutrients.

Current dietary guidelines for phytonutrients recommend seven servings of fresh fruits and vegetables per day. Obviously many of us—especially those who do not follow the **Say Yes to NO Plan**—do not even come close to meeting this requirement through our diet. The good news is that many nutritional supplement companies today are producing *fruit and vegetable phytonutrient supplements*. You may have heard of some of the important phytonutrients contained in these supplements, including:

Lycopene: a powerful antioxidant found in the red pigment of tomatoes. Lycopene helps prevent cardiovascular disease and several types of cancer.

Lutein and Zeaxanthin: carotenoids found in dark green, leafy vegetables like spinach, avocado, collard greens, and green peas. Lutein and zeaxanthin specifically target the eyes, reducing the risk of macular degeneration and retinal damage.

Allicin: contained in garlic. Allicin has multiple benefits for the immune system, it helps reduce cholesterol, and it supports the health of the digestive system.

Grapes: antioxidant effects are due to an array of polyphenol phytonutrients like resveratrol, anthocyanins, catechins, quercetin. The phytonutrients in grapes are at the bottom of the "French Paradox," in which drinking moderate amounts of wine and/or grape juice has been shown to protect the heart and blood vessels against oxidative tissue damage.

Bioflavonoids: antioxidants found in many fruits and vegetables, including apricots, blackberries, broccoli, cherries, grapefruits, grapes, oranges, and lemons. Bioflavonoids work closely with vitamin C, helping prevent vitamin C from being oxidized. They have also been shown to stop or slow the growth of malignant cells, as well as protect against cancer-causing substances that invade the cardiovascular system.

Broccoli sprout extract: along with other plants from the brassica family, contains the phytonutrient sulforaphane. Sulforaphane mobilizes a set of enzymes that neutralize highly reactive cancer-causing chemicals before they damage DNA and promote cancer.

Do whatever you can to eat at least seven servings each day of the foods—a wide range of fruits and vegetables—that contain these critical phytonutrients. They not only work to improve your overall health, but either directly or indirectly they support your body's production of nitric oxide.

Here is some of the research that proves fiber is a NO–guarding antioxidant:

- In research published in the *American Journal of Cardiology* in 1992, Stanford University investigators examined the effects of increasing amounts of soluble fiber on blood cholesterol levels. They found that individuals with elevated cholesterol readings (above 200 mg/dl) who consumed 5 grams of soluble fiber per day for four weeks reduced their LDL ("bad") cholesterol by 5.6 percent. The reductions were much more impressive when the amount of soluble fiber rose to

15 grams, which caused LDL levels to plummet by 14.9 percent.

- At the University of Minnesota Medical School, researchers compared people with high blood pressure who were placed on high-fiber oat cereals versus those in a control group consuming low-fiber cereals for six weeks. As reported in the *Journal of Family Practice* in 2002, those volunteers eating the high-fiber cereal experienced an average 7.5 mm Hg reduction in their systolic blood pressure and a 5.5 mm Hg decline in their diastolic blood pressure, compared to virtually no change among the controls. The high-fiber group also showed significant declines in their total cholesterol (9 percent) and LDL cholesterol (14 percent).

There is another significant cardiovascular plus to high-fiber foods. They tend to contain other nutrients like vitamin C and vitamin E, powerful antioxidants that stimulate your production of NO!

Fiber and L-Arginine

In Avellino, Italy, investigators at the Institute of Food Sciences and Technology performed a study using six healthy volunteers with an average age of thirty-nine, published in 2000 in the *American Journal of Hypertension*. These individuals were placed on a sequence of three diets, assigned in random order, each for a one-week duration.

RESULTS OF L-ARGININE STUDY

Diet	Description of Diet	Results
Diet 1	Control diet: 3.5–4.0 grams L-arginine per day	Control
Diet 2	More L-arginine rich foods: 10 grams L-arginine per day	Blood pressure lower than control by 6.2 mm Hg systolic and 5.0 mm Hg diastolic. Improved total cholesterol and HDL cholesterol, as well as triglyceride levels.
Diet 3	Supplement: Diet 1 plus an oral supplement to total 10 grams L-arginine per day	Blood pressure lower than control by 6.2 mm Hg systolic and 6.8 mm Hg diastolic.

The conclusions from the study are clear: The addition of L-arginine, whether in functional foods or supplement form, caused a significant decrease in blood pressure. Diet 2, which included functional foods rich in L-arginine, also showed improvements in cholesterol and triglyceride levels, while the supplement-based Diet 3 did not. The researchers hypothesized that this difference could be related to the higher fiber composition of Diet 2. While more work is being done in this area, the combination of boosting L-arginine and increasing your fiber consumption is one that you should consider—and which will result from your adherence to the **Say Yes to NO Plan.**

Jumping on the Fiber Bandwagon

- If your are boosting your dietary fiber for the first time, you can reduce the gas and bloating that sometimes accompany increases in fiber intake by adding these foods to your diet very gradually. Your eventual aim each day should be around 25 grams of fiber.

- Make sure to drink eight glasses of water a day.

- Choose whole grain, whole wheat breads and cereals (particularly bran cereals and oatmeal) with at least 3 grams of fiber.

- Sprinkle bran on your morning cereal, on salads, and in meat loaf as well as home-baked muffins and breads.

- Getting your fiber from foods is preferable to getting it from supplements.

- All types of beans and peas are particularly good sources of fiber.

- All types of nuts and seeds are particularly good sources of fiber.

- Vegetables and fruits lose considerable fiber when pureed, so steam them or eat them raw.

A high-fiber diet can serve as an adjunct to the other strategies described in this book, all targeted to the successful management of your risk of cardiovascular disease.

FISH AND SEAFOOD: OUR CARDIOVASCULAR GIFTS FROM THE SEA

One source of healthy fat has been recognized by cardiologists—namely, seafood. Most fish have low levels of saturated fat, and in many cases, high amounts of omega-3 fatty acids, an oil that is an ally of your cardiovascular health.

Omega-3 fatty acids from fish oils help reduce total blood fats, reduce LDL (bad) cholesterol, and raise HDL (good) cholesterol. In addition, fish oils benefit the heart by keeping platelets, saturated fats, and cholesterol from sticking together and clogging arteries, contributing to heart attack and stroke.

A published research study showed that one serving of salmon per week can cut the risk of heart attack in half. Researchers in another study followed more than 20,000 male physicians between forty and eighty years of age for eleven years and observed the amount of fish consumed. The results showed that the physicians who ate fish once a week were 52 percent less likely to die of a fatal cardiac arrhythmia (irregular heart beat) than those who consumed fish only once a month.

The Alaskan Paradox

For many years, researchers were puzzled by the fact that the Eskimos of Greenland and the Native Americans in Alaska ate a substantial amount of whale blubber and seal meat and had very little heart disease. Finally, they were able to solve the mystery. Among the fats in seal meat and whale blubber is a profusion of heart-healthy omega-3 fatty acids, which work to maintain low blood pressure and LDL cholesterol, while encouraging the body's natural production of HDL and discouraging the formation of plaque and blood clots in the cardiovascular system.

Omega-3 and NO

There is now strong evidence that fish can reduce your level of *triglycerides*—natural fats and oils which, when overabundant in the bloodstream, seem to be linked to atherosclerosis, heart attack, and stroke. A growing body of research indicates that if you eat fish two to three times a week, you will significantly reduce your risk of heart disease—and not only because of its effects on triglycerides.

Fish oils can protect your endothelial cells—and their ability to make NO—by interfering with the oxidation process, blocking platelet aggregation that can trigger a heart attack or stroke, and even minimizing the risk of heart arrhythmias. In a study published in 1997 in *Biochemical and Biophysical Research Communications,* Japanese researchers at the University of Tsukuba joined other scientific teams who have conducted laboratory in vitro research that has consistently shown that the production of NO increased within minutes after exposure to omega-3 fatty acids.

Fish and Shellfish: Foods Your Heart Loves

If you do not presently eat fish often, please introduce it frequently into your diet. The variety of types of fish and shellfish is so great, you are bound to find a few selections that appeal to you. I am a big fan of sushi, which provides many heart-healthy benefits: omega-3s from the fish, antioxidants in the soy sauce, and vitamins C and E in the nori. Nori is seaweed, which now appears to play an important role in reducing high blood pressure, along with other common cardiovascular conditions.

The highest levels of omega-3 fatty acids are found in cold-water marine fish, including:

Salmon

Tuna

Mackerel (also contains a substantial amount of fats, including saturated fat; if you have cardiovascular problems, salmon or tuna would be a better choice)

Herring

Halibut

Sardines

Seafood is also a heart-healthy source of low-fat protein. Remember, amino acids—among them L-arginine and L-citrulline—are the building blocks of protein, and they are known to encourage your body's production of nitric oxide. The best sources of protein in seafood are:

Tuna

Salmon

Snapper

Swordfish

Lobster

Shrimp

Cod

When it comes to eating fish, pregnant and lactating women should exercise caution. Studies in recent years show some fish contain high levels of mercury and PCBs, which are dangerous to fetuses and young children. It is best for these women to avoid excess intake of swordfish, shark, king mackerel, tile fish, and albacore tuna (but not the "chunk light" variety that comes in a can).

The Truth about Shellfish and Cholesterol

I am sure you have heard that shellfish is dangerously high in cholesterol and should be avoided by people with high LDL cholesterol levels. Actually, the LDL cholesterol content of certain shellfish, like lobster and crab meat, is as low as or lower than that of skinless white meat of chicken or lean beef. If you have preexisting cardiovascular problems, you might want to eat shrimp (which contains 160 mg of LDL cholesterol per three-ounce serving) and squid (with 233 mg of LDL cholesterol) infrequently. If your "bad" cholesterol is high, you might want to restrict your shellfish meals to two or three times a week—just to be on the safe side.

Taking the Supplement Route

If you are allergic to seafood or just cannot stomach it, there is another way to incorporate more fish oils in your diet. Fish oil capsules, available in most health food stores, contain omega-3 fatty acids and can help maintain your endothelial health. Study results have been mixed on whether these supplements are as effective as eating fish itself. I recommend incorporating at least some fish into your diet.

Eggs: They're Not Just for Bodybuilders Any More

Eggs have long been known to be a good source of NO-boosting protein, but they are not without their downside—the high levels of LDL or "bad" cholesterol contained in the yolk. The solution is simple: Avoid the bad cholesterol in whole eggs and eat instead only the protein-rich whites. Almost all restaurants offer a wide variety of egg-white omelets that are tasty and heart-healthy.

Nuts Pack a Protein Punch

Nuts—soybeans, hazelnuts, walnuts, almonds, and peanuts—are a tremendous protein package that also contain a substance to enhance vascular relaxation. Recently it has been shown that a judicious snack of nuts before mealtime can actually decrease the appetite—making nuts a terrific aid to dieters. They are also great for vegans. When crushed, nuts are great as a crust on fish and chicken. They are flavorful additions to your morning cereal as well as important contributors to delicious yet good-for-you treats like date-nut bread.

GO FOR THE GARLIC

The therapeutic uses of garlic date back to India 5,000 years ago, where it was used to clean wounds, even to help fight off colds, and kill invading bacteria. It was not until recently that we discovered why garlic heals. When garlic is crushed or sliced, it releases a sulphurous compound called *allicin,* which gives it not only its pungent odor but also its curative abilities, because it is a powerful antioxidant.

Garlic and NO

Science has focused on garlic's ability to lower cholesterol and blood pressure and to help guard your body against stroke and heart disease. We are coming around to thinking that garlic's efficiency in preventing stroke and heart disease is because it acts against depressed NO production, improving cardiovascular function in the process.

The Observer Food Monthly magazine reports that "when the *Journal of the Royal College of Physicians* reviewed data on cholesterol in 1993, it found that after just four weeks there was a twelve per cent reduction in cholesterol levels in the research groups that had taken garlic."

The same publication also tells us that "a review of recent clinical trials, published in the *Journal of Hypertension,* showed that taking garlic tablets cut volunteers' blood pressure by between 1 and 5 percent. These results led the report's authors to conclude that taking supplements could cut the incidence of stroke by 30 to 40 percent, while heart disease could be reduced by 20 to 25 percent."

How Much Garlic Should You Take a Day—and in What Form?

If you are taking an anticoagulant, pregnant, or breast-feeding, garlic could possibly have a deleterious effect, so do not take it.

The rest of us have many choices: fresh cloves, capsules, pills, or tablets, or juice.

Fresh cloves: One to three cloves per day.
Capsules, pills, and tablets: If you cannot stand what fresh garlic does to your breath or if it gives you indigestion, you should be taking 300 mg, two to three times a day.
Juice: 20 to 30 drops per day.

Since garlic as an antioxidant appears to increase NO production, it could be a potent weapon in your war against cardiovascular disease. Why not try it?

GREEN TEA WORKS CARDIOVASCULAR MAGIC

Green tea has been known in China as a powerful healing agent for at least 4000 years. More recently medical researchers can begin to explain why green tea seems to be effective against:

Cancer—especially prostate and breast cancer
Rheumatoid arthritis
High blood pressure
High LDL cholesterol
Atherosclerosis
Blood clots
Heart attack
Stroke

By the way, green tea also seems to speed up the rate at which the body burns up fat, making its consumption supportive of weight loss.

Green Tea's Secret Weapon and NO

We now know that green tea contains a major antioxidant called EGCG (epigallocatechin gallate), which appears to kill cancer cells without harming healthy ones, to provide smokers with a shield against heart disease, and to improve cardiovascular health. EGCG as an antioxidant combats oxidative stress and in so doing, protects your endothelial cells from invading molecules, thereby safeguarding NO production.

Who Shouldn't Take Green Tea?

Green tea does contain caffeine, so if your doctor has taken you off coffee because of a medical condition like ulcers or high blood pressure, check with him before beginning green tea therapy.

What Is the Recommended Dosage for Green Tea?

As a Supplement: 250–500 mg per day

As a Tea: One to three cups brewed with a teaspoon of leaf daily

FLAXSEED: A *VERY* GOOD THING

The flax plant has been known to civilization from ancient times, because its fibers are woven into linen. Now we know flaxseed is an important player in maintaining cardiovascular health. Its seeds can be left whole and chewed, or made into meal or an oil. Whatever form you choose will do wonders for your cardiovascular health.

Flaxseed and NO

The often overlooked fiber-rich grain called flaxseed is one of the best antioxidants in your nutritional arsenal. Flaxseed oil is loaded with omega-3 fatty acids and soluble fiber. It has a startling 53 grams of omega-3s per 3.5 ounces of the oil, compared to 11 grams in an equal amount of canola oil. You will remember, omega-3s are dedicated to protecting your endothelial cells against the invasion of free radicals—guaranteeing that nitric oxide will continue to be produced at heart-healthy levels.

How to Use Flaxseed to Your Heart's Content

You can buy flaxseed oil in bottles, but I generally recommend looking for flaxseed in its other formulations. The oil on grocery store shelves may already be oxidized, and it will not provide all the benefits of flaxseed. I suggest that you go to a whole foods market and purchase a one-pound bag of real flaxseed. It is very inexpensive. The seeds do not need to be refrigerated as long as the shells are on them. Grind a little of it in a coffee bean grinder used exclusively for flaxseed. Once it has been ground into a powder, sprinkle about two tablespoons of it on a bowl of high-fiber breakfast cereal or on a salad. Fully 100 percent of the flaxseed oil is liberated this way. It tastes great, and it has a wonderfully fresh smell. If you spend time in the kitchen, you can also try baking bread with flaxseed in it.

If you look at the research on the positive effects of flaxseed on cholesterol levels, much of it was conducted at the Kenneth L. Jordan Heart Foundation and Research Center in Montclair, New Jersey, where volunteers consumed their flaxseed in bread. In one of those studies, published in the *Journal of the American College of Nutrition* in 1993, fifteen people with high blood cholesterol levels (averaging 266 mg/dl) ate three slices of flaxseed-enriched bread per day; the flaxseed made up 10 percent of the weight of every loaf. These men and women also consumed another 15 grams of ground flaxseed each day. When their cholesterol was measured after three months on this flaxseed regimen, their total cholesterol levels had dropped significantly from 266 to 248 mg/dl, while their LDL cholesterol dipped from 190 to 171 mg/dl.

THE SOY PHENOMENON

Not too many years ago, most Americans had probably never tasted soy. That still may be the case. Even so, the word is beginning to spread about soy's benefits, and more people are consuming it in everything from soy burgers to soy milk, from tofu to tempeh.

Soy and NO

Soy has been a staple of the diet in Japan for many years with a substantial payoff. As you may know, heart disease is much lower—and the lifespan is longer—among the Japanese than it is among Americans, and at least part of the credit belongs to soy. The Japanese diet tends to be higher in fiber and lower in fat than ours, and soybeans make a big difference. Soy is filled with phytonutrients that function as antioxidants and fight everything from cardiovascular disease to cancers of the breast and prostate. In particular, soy substances called *isoflavones* interfere with the oxidation of blood fats, preventing free radicals from being formed and from causing endothelial damage that interferes with NO production.

Soy: A Triple Threat to High Cholesterol

A growing number of nutritionists and scientists are finding themselves persuaded by the mounting evidence supporting a role for soy in a heart-healthy diet. In 2001, for example, researchers at the University of Milano in Italy wrote, "The soybean diet is the most potent dietary tool for hypercholesterolemia [high cholesterol levels]." In *Current Atherosclerosis Reports*, they pointed to a number of hypotheses explaining how soy may reduce cholesterol levels, including its rich content of phytoestrogens, its soy fiber, and even the soy protein itself.

At the University of Kentucky, researchers reviewed thirty-eight studies that examined the influence of soy protein upon the cholesterol levels of a total of 740 men and women. In the *New England Journal of Medicine* in 1995, the scientists reported that when eating an average of 47 grams of soy protein a day rather than animal protein, total cholesterol levels dipped 9.3 percent, LDL cholesterol declined 12.9 percent, and triglycerides fell 10.5 percent. At the same time, HDL cholesterol levels climbed 2.4 percent, although this increase was not statistically significant.

Getting the Max from Dietary Soy

There are plenty of ways to incorporate soy into your diet. Try whole soy yogurt; you cannot beat the taste. Or use soy milk. Add soy to your diet with miso soup, roasted soy nuts, tempeh, soy flour, tofu, and soy burgers and franks—as well as salmon teriyaki, sushi, and sashimi. Recently edamame—soybeans in the pod—has become popular as a tasty snack, thanks to the many sushi restaurants that serve it. You can buy frozen edamame at most health food stores.

Soy is too good for you to pass up!

THE BRIGHT SIDE OF DARK CHOCOLATE

You may not believe it yet, but chocolate is good for your cardiovascular health.

Chocolate—specifically dark chocolate and cocoa powder—can boost your levels of NO. Dark chocolate and cocoa powder are rich in the antioxidants that send free radicals to their deaths, protecting NO production, which results in the relaxation of blood vessels. Relaxed blood vessels in turn lower blood pressure, raise HDL cholesterol, and help protect you from heart attack and stroke.

Chocolate and NO

Saturated fat—usually a menace to your cardiovascular system—is an ingredient in chocolate, but the precise types of saturated fat—called *stearic acid* and *palmitic acid*—are actually innocuous, inert, and not detrimental to your heart. Carefully conducted studies at the University of Texas Southwestern Medical School in Dallas found that, unlike most other saturated fats, stearic acid has a neutral effect on blood cholesterol levels and cardiovascular health. It is simply eliminated from the body.

The benefits of chocolate and cocoa powder rest with substances called *polyphenols,* which are antioxidants that can minimize free radical damage and preserve NO. The following research findings show the benefits:

- A study by researchers at Brigham and Women's Hospital and Harvard Medical School looked at the antioxidant properties of cocoa. Their data, presented at the American Association for the Advancement of Science meeting in 2002, showed that the antioxidants in cocoa actually appear to support nitric oxide synthesis.

- A study at the University of California, Davis, evaluated the effects of an antioxidant-rich cocoa beverage in thirty healthy subjects. In their study in the *American Journal of Clinical Nutrition* in 2000, they concluded that the cocoa drink reduced blood platelet activity and aggregation, similar to an aspirinlike effect, thus lowering the risk of blood clotting.

- In a study at Pennsylvania State University, published in the *American Journal of Clinical Nutrition* in 2001, researchers gave twenty-three men and women a diet containing half an ounce of dark chocolate and an ounce of cocoa powder. After four weeks, they concluded that the cocoa/dark chocolate diet interfered with the oxidation of LDL cholesterol. It reduced oxidation to about an 8 percent slower rate than in controls. HDL cholesterol levels were 4 percent higher on the chocolate diet.

Many people prefer sweet milk chocolate to the dark variety—and I admit that dark chocolate can seem somewhat bitter. You are incorporating chocolate into your diet not to indulge your sweet tooth, but for the antioxidants, and milk chocolate does not have any of the antioxidants in dark chocolate, because they are all lost in the processing.

Moderation, Moderation, Moderation

Probably the biggest drawback to dark chocolate is that it contains plenty of calories. My advice is to consume chocolate only in moderation. If you enjoy chocolate, and want to have a few pieces each day as a snack, choose dark chocolate. Consume no more than about 120 calories of dark chocolate in any given day. Divide it in small pieces and eat them throughout the afternoon and evening, one bite at a time.

One other caveat: As the Pennsylvania State University researchers pointed out in their published paper cited above, dark chocolate can increase your antioxidant intake, but it is only one means of doing so. Chocolate should be consumed prudently and sensibly as only a small part of an overall healthy diet that includes fruits, vegetables, whole grains, reduced-fat dairy products, fatty fish, lean meat, and poultry.

RED WINE: BEYOND THE FRENCH PARADOX

Maybe you have heard of the French paradox. For years, it has been a mystery why the people of France can eat a high-fat diet without many consequences—consuming plenty of rich cheeses and butter-drenched croissants, while smoking cigarettes so zealously that they leave most American visitors gasping for fresh air. Even so, their rates of heart disease are markedly lower than those found in the United States. It is an intriguing phenomenon, and it continues to baffle cardiologists.

The missing link in the mystery may rest with the popularity of wine in France. The French consume much more wine per capita than Americans do, and there is growing evidence that the ingredients of wine may be protective of the heart.

Red Wine and NO

Wine consumption, of course, has a history that dates back thousands of years, but only relatively recently have scientists started looking carefully at its medicinal benefits. Initially, researchers were impressed by large epidemiological studies showing that people who drank a glass or two of wine a day had a greater life expectancy, and were less likely to develop heart disease.

Scientists began studying the specific ingredients of wine under the microscope. They found that red wine in particular is rich in polyphenols—antioxidants that interfere with platelet aggregation and also appear to protect nitric oxide and markedly stimulate NO production. Wine and other types of alcohol can also increase the levels of HDL cholesterol in the blood and may interfere with the inflammatory processes that can contribute to heart disease.

A Word of Warning

Before you pop the cork on a bottle of Bordeaux, cabernet sauvignon, or pinot noir and figure that you have finally won the war against heart disease, I do not recommend red wine for everyone. If you already enjoy a glass of wine with dinner, red wine seems an excellent choice because of its rich antioxidant content. Just remember to keep your red wine intake at a moderate level—no more than a glass or two a day. If you do not already drink, do not start. Despite the impressive benefits of red wine, the risks associated with alcohol use in general—from alcoholism to life-threatening liver problems—are too serious for me to recommend that teetotalers start drinking.

GRAPE JUICE IS BIG MEDICINE

If you have decided to leave the red wine to the Europeans, there appears to be another simple way to reap many of its benefits in a rather innocuous way. You may find that purple grape juice works just as well. Grape juice contains the same polyphenols that are found in red wine; it just has not been fermented.

Grape Juice and NO

At Georgetown University, volunteers were asked to drink about two cups of purple grape juice a day for two weeks. In a study published in *Circulation* in 2001, the researchers reported that the consumption of grape juice increased the levels of vitamin E (alpha-tocopherol) in their plasma by 13 percent, and elevated their nitric oxide production from platelets by a full 70 percent. At the same time, the overall platelet activity in their blood declined significantly, reducing the likelihood of blood clots.

Whether or not red wine ever becomes part of your life, you might start stocking the cupboard with purple grape juice.

BLUEBERRIES RULE THE ROOST

If you are looking for a potent source of antioxidants, you cannot do much better than blueberries. Blueberries are believed to function by preserving the bioavailabilty of nitric oxide.

Blueberries and NO

In a recent study at the U.S. Department of Agriculture Human Nutrition Research Center on Aging at Tufts University, blueberries were ranked as the best source of antioxidant activity and NO protection when compared to forty other fruits and vegetables—better than strawberries, better than kale, better than garlic, spinach, and every other food that was tested. They are also a good source of fiber. Blueberries contain plenty of pectin, which may be best known as a cholesterol-lowering fiber found in apples, most other fruits, and many vegetables.

POMEGRANATE JUICE: THE UP AND COMER

Recent studies in Israel have shown that pomegranate juice may be vying to be the richest known source of natural antioxidants—possessing more healthful polyphenols than red wine and green tea. The juice from pomegranates can not only protect against increases in cholesterol levels in humans, but it can also actually lower cholesterol counts. In animal studies, pomegranate juice effectively reduced the severity of atherosclerosis.

Pomegranate Juice and NO

The polyphenols in pomegranate juice are powerful antioxidants, protecting NO production and boosting cardiovascular wellness. In one recent study, people who drank just two ounces a day for a week increased antioxidant activity by 9 percent.

If you are not familiar with pomegranate juice, give it a try. It has a unique, pleasant taste.

A LIFESTYLE SHIFT YOU'LL THANK ME FOR

I hope you will try combining the dietary suggestions mentioned in this chapter with the supplements you read about in Chapter 6. As you do, your levels of NO should rise significantly, thus reducing your risk of cardiovascular disease. In a matter of weeks, I expect you to be feeling great!

Say Yes to NO—Simply Awesome!

"I've been following Dr. Ignarro's NO-boosting recommendations for supplements, nutrition, and exercise for about a week. I noticed right away that my coloring had improved and my skin was even-toned. I also get 'jolts' of 'rejuvenation' throughout the day. It is awesome. I can feel my insides literally being replenished. What an unbelievable feeling!"

Teri, 37, Buffalo

In the following chapter, we will take the next step—adding moderate amounts of exercise to your lifestyle as another way to protect the health of your heart.

THE HEART OF THE MATTER

Before we move on, let's review what you have learned in this chapter.

- By reducing your intake of saturated fat, you will protect your endothelium and its ability to manufacture nitric oxide.

- An increase in your consumption of dietary fiber can help reduce your risk of coronary artery disease.

- Fish and shellfish contain omega-3 fatty acids, which interfere with the oxidation process, and in turn, facilitate NO production. Flaxseed is another good source of omega-3s.

- Garlic contains the sulfurous compound *allicin,* which is the source of both garlic's pungent odor and its powerful antioxidant qualities.

- Soy is filled with antioxidant chemicals that prevent the formation of oxygen radicals.

- Dark chocolate is rich in polyphenols, which are a type of antioxidant that can minimize oxidative damage and protect nitric oxide. In addition, red wine, purple grape juice, pomegranate juice, and blueberries are other excellent sources of polyphenols.

8

SAY YES TO NO-BOOSTING FITNESS

I am a great believer in the adage, "Make the time to exercise now, or you'll be forced to take a break from your life in five, ten, or twenty years when you end up in a hospital bed."

There is a clear payoff to being physically active, and it is called good health. If you are one of those people whose physical activity has been confined to rushing from one business meeting to the next, or pushing a shopping cart down the aisles of the local supermarket, I hope this chapter will convince you that you are doing your body a severe disservice.

I am only asking for twenty minutes of your time. As busy as your life is, you can find twenty minutes, at least three times a week, to devote to exercise, can't you? Everyone can. Even if you do not exercise every day, your endothelial health will be strengthened and maintained if you can maintain a workout schedule of three to four times a week. At that activity level, your workouts are training your endothelial cells to make additional NO continuously—even on days when you are not exercising.

Take Heart—with NO-Boosting Exercise

A 1996 German study at the University of Freiburg put people with chronic heart failure on a daily half-hour program of light physical training for a month. Researchers subsequently concluded that, as the result of the exercise regimen, the subjects' vessels began functioning better. The reason, they hypothesized, was most likely related to exercise-induced increases in the release of NO.

Once you become a regular exerciser, you will literally begin to "train" your endothelial cells to make more NO even when you are not working out. Exercise is the only known process that causes a consistent and continuous production of NO by the endothelial cells, long after you have done your last sit-up or taken your last step on the treadmill for the day.

THE NO/FITNESS FACTOR: LOWERING BLOOD PRESSURE AND CHOLESTEROL, REDUCING ARTERIAL PLAQUE

Blood Pressure

For years, cardiologists have urged patients with hypertension to exercise, because physical activity tends to result in a reduction of dosages of hypertensive medication, often eliminating the need for them completely, as well as a decline in blood pressure. Now we know why. Exercise can help ensure that your endothelial cells are producing sufficient amounts of

NO, which keeps your blood flow cruising, rather than racing, through the body.

Cholesterol

Exercise can aid in improving your cholesterol level. Physical activity can raise the blood levels of the "good" HDL cholesterol. When it comes to your HDL, the higher the better. NO is a key factor in exercise's ability to readjust your cholesterol profile in a positive way by influencing the genes that control the fats in the blood. A growing body of research shows that regular exercise can boost HDL levels by a full 5 to 15 percent.

It might interest you to know that in a Brigham Young University study published in the *American Journal of Public Health,* researchers evaluated the effects of regular walking on the cholesterol profiles of more than 3,600 adults. Those individuals who walked for 2.5 to 4 (or more) hours per week were more likely to have a cholesterol ratio (total cholesterol-to-HDL cholesterol) that was favorable (a ratio of 5.0 or lower) than a group who did not exercise regularly. This cholesterol ratio, of course, is one of the most frequently used indicators of your cardiovascular disease risk.

Arterial Plaque

When plaque builds up on the walls of your arteries, these fatty deposits can impede the normal flow of blood and increase the likelihood of blockages within the vessels. When arterial plaque happens, heart attack or stroke is likely to follow. Exercise-enhanced nitric oxide production can help, since NO discourages blood platelets from sticking to the inner lining of the vessels and reduces the risk of plaque accumulation and blood clots.

If you can keep your endothelial cells extra-healthy with NO-generating exercise, they can continue to protect the vessels and lower your chances of developing atherosclerosis.

Conquering the Elements

"I bicycle up to fifty miles per week in the hot Las Vegas sun. Since starting NO therapy, the endurance in my legs and ability to withstand the heat this summer has been amazing. The only thing that stops me is the amount of water I can carry and the padding on my seat!"

Steve, 33, Las Vegas

NO PLUS—A RANGE OF FITNESS BENEFITS

Physical activity seems to produce additional positive health results that appear not to be directly related to nitric oxide, but being in great cardiovascular shape makes you an excellent candidate for any and all fitness benefits:

- Regular exercise can strengthen your heart and make it work more efficiently. Since your muscles need more oxygen when you are active, your heart has to pump more vigorously to transport blood to every region of the body. Over time, as the heart becomes stronger, it is able to deliver more blood with each beat, and your resting heart rate will become lower.

- Exercise can put you on the fast track toward weight loss. Obesity is an epidemic in the U.S.; according to the Centers for Disease Control and Prevention, an alarming 97 million adult Americans are overweight or obese. At any given time, 35 to 40 percent of women, and 20 to 24 percent of men, are dieting. Yet many of them do not see exercise as part of that weight-loss equation.

My Personal Best

"Nitric oxide therapy helped me to improve my marathon run by forty-one minutes. I ran the marathon last year and my time was 5:16. This year, my time improved to 4:35, despite the fact that I'm one year older (fifty-eight). **Say Yes to NO** helps me run better every day and sleep better every night!"

Chris, 58, San Francisco

Here is some advice: Whether you are trying to lose a few—or quite a few—pounds, nothing can expend calories quicker than regular exercise (thirty minutes of walking burns about 200 calories). Physical activity accelerates your metabolism, and not only while you are exercising. Your metabolism works overtime even after you have worked out. Some research shows that your metabolic rate remains elevated for up to several hours following your workout. The more strenuous and prolonged the exercise session, the longer the metabolism continues to burn calories before returning to its resting level. Add to that the ability of exercise to preserve and increase lean muscle mass, decrease your body fat percentage, and put a damper on your appetite—and you have even more reasons to keep moving. In addition, people who are physically active experience:

- A lower risk of breast, prostate, and colon cancer.

- An increase in insulin sensitivity and an improvement in carbohydrate metabolism. These changes reduce your risk of developing type II (adult-onset) diabetes.

- A reduced likelihood of developing osteoporosis, the bone thinning disease that affects millions of post-menopausal women as well as many men. Weight-bearing exercise like walking can keep your bones strong, even increasing your bone density.

- A decline in stress and anxiety levels.

- An improved overall sense of well-being. Some researchers believe that this improved mental state is related to hormones called endorphins, which are the body's own tranquilizer or antidepressant and which tend to increase in number during and after exercise.

- A stronger disease-fighting immune system.

- Greater energy levels.

- Improved quality of sleep.

Cardiovascular Age-Proofing: A Proven Fact

In a paper published in the journal *Circulation* in 2000, Italian researchers examined whether the impairment of the endothelium—which has been described as part of the aging process—can be minimized by regular physical activity. They evaluated the health of the endothelial cells in older people (average age sixty-four years) who exercised, compared with those of much younger individuals (average age twenty-eight years). The older exercisers had blood vessels that were as healthy and functional as those of the younger group. The researchers concluded that "regular physical training protects the vascular endothelium from aging-related alterations." This positive effect of exercise, they added, is "related to preservation of NO availability."

AS YOU LIKE IT: CUSTOMIZING YOUR WORKOUT ROUTINE

Unfortunately, as people age, most of them tend to become more sedentary, and perhaps pay a little less attention to their diet as well. Those kinds of lifestyle changes can contribute to a decline in your body's production of NO, which can only accelerate the aging process. Exercise cannot stop the march of time, but it can make you physiologically younger than people your same age who are sedentary.

If you are part of the sedentary masses, it is time for a major change. If you are worried that you are going to need to start running marathons or make the local gym your home away from home, you can relax. Most research now shows that you do not have to exercise to the point of exhaustion to achieve the NO–related benefits of an active lifestyle. All you need is a commitment to exercise at a moderate level, and to do it regularly.

NO Dispensed with His Workout Pain

"I go to the local gym four days a week and work out for two hours each time with free weights. I noticed that after three weeks of NO therapy, the pains in my arms and legs accompanying or following my workouts disappeared. This was truly a miraculous find!"

Paul, 35, Los Angeles

I recommend selecting a type of exercise that improves your aerobic fitness. That means choosing an activity that forces you to breathe deeply and continuously for at least twenty minutes, using major muscle groups and giving your cardiovascular system a good workout. There are plenty of options that fall into this category. For example:

- Walking
- Jogging
- Bicycling
- Swimming
- Tennis
- Squash
- Basketball
- Yoga
- Pilates
- Cross-country skiing
- Jumping rope
- Rollerblading (in-line skating)

- Rowing
- Gardening
- Dancing

My Minimum Prescription for Exercise: Twenty Minutes, Three Days a Week

I talk about many different aspects of exercise in this chapter, giving you plenty of options of what to do and how to do it. But I want to be clear—the bottom line minimum you should be shooting for in your NO-boosting workout regimen is twenty minutes, three days a week. If your current fitness level is quite low, you may have to work slowly to reach this level, but it is where you ultimately want to be—at a minimum.

Once you have reached the minimum level—and perhaps you are already there or beyond as you read this—you can decide whether or not to continue and strive for even greater benefits. My prediction is that you will, because the great feelings exercise gives your body and mind can be addicting—as are the additional long-term health benefits that a more extensive program can provide.

Clearly there are many different ways of getting a moderate to strenuous NO-boosting aerobic workout doing something you enjoy. My customized workout concentrates on walking. Hippocrates described walking as "man's best medicine." Virtually anyone can walk, no matter what his or her age or fitness level. Walking is simple. You do not need to hire a personal trainer to teach you to walk. You will not have to invest in any special equipment, although I do strongly recommend buying a good pair of walking shoes. You can walk briskly or at a slower rate, but over time, as your muscle mass increases and your lung capacity improves, try picking up the pace.

The Walking Cure

In 1994, two groups of sedentary British women (average age forty-seven) participated in a study seeking to find a link between physical activity and increased health benefits. One group adopted a brisk walking program for twelve weeks, while the other remained sedentary. Not surprisingly, the active women showed significant increases in their "good" cholesterol. When the active group stopped their walking regimen and were retested six months later, their cholesterol improvement had regressed.

Some people alternate activities to avoid boredom. For example, they will walk for half of their workouts and swim for the other half. Or if walking drives them to tears, they will read or watch TV while pedaling an exercise bicycle. Or they put on some earphones and let music keep them company during their workout. Too many home exercise machines have been collecting dust in America's closets, or they have been turned into rather expensive clothing racks, because of the boredom experienced by their owners.

If It Isn't Fun, Don't Do It!

One of the most valuable pieces of advice I can give you is to choose a type of exercise that you enjoy. If you are having fun exercising, you're much more likely to stick with it, one day after another, one week after the next. That is the key to reaping the full benefits of physical activity. Regular, consistent exercise is crucial to your well-being. On the other hand, if you choose an exercise that you consider to be absolute drudgery—and if you have to force yourself to do it—it is almost inevitable that your exercise program is doomed.

MAKE SAY YES TO NO FITNESS A HABIT!

There are times when you are faced with a particularly unforgiving deadline at work, or a demanding schedule, and you will miss a day of exercise here or there. As much as possible schedule your NO-boosting workouts just as you would any other appointment, and consider it just as important as almost anything else in your life. Exercise is not an optional activity; it is a necessity.

When you travel, pack your workout clothes and stay in hotels that have exercise rooms. Abandoning your exercise program when you go on the road would be like leaving your medicine bottles at home if you were taking blood-pressure pills. If you are a diabetic, you take your insulin with you wherever you go. You should do the same with **Say Yes To NO** Fitness.

GO SLOWLY—THE GOLDEN RULE OF EXERCISE

You do not have to set any world records to enjoy the benefits of exercise. Do your workout activity at a moderate, comfortable pace. If you would like, check your pulse periodically. For someone of average fitness level, aim for 110 to 120 beats a minute. You can stop and count heartbeats if you would like, but here is an easier rule of thumb: If you cannot carry on a conversation while you are performing your exercise, you are probably moving too fast. If that happens, slow down a little. Overexerting yourself and gasping for your next breath is not going to motivate you to keep exercise as a regular part of your life. Nor will you generate any extra NO by boosting your heart rate beyond 120.

In fact, going too hard and too fast could actually be hazardous to your health. If you push your body to the limit, exercise can cause an overproduction of free radicals, which can undermine your well-being and counteract the benefits of working out. If you have been diagnosed with coronary artery disease, do not aim for maximum exertion. If you get the blood flowing through your arteries at full force, you could dislodge plaques from the vessel walls and trigger a heart attack.

Working Out Saves Lives

One of the most revealing studies about exercise intensity was conducted at the Institute for Aerobics Research. In landmark research published in the *Journal of the*

American Medical Association in 1989, more than 13,000 men and women were given treadmill tests, and then their fitness levels and health status were monitored for the next eight years. Those people who got no exercise at all had a greater risk of developing chronic diseases and dying prematurely—with a death rate more than three times higher than the individuals who exercised the most.

The researchers arrived at a rather unexpected conclusion. They discovered that the individuals who experienced some of the greatest health benefits from exercise were those who simply walked thirty minutes a day, three to four times a week. These moderate exercisers lowered their risk of premature death nearly as much as the people who ran thirty to forty miles a week, with only slight differences in the mortality rates among these exercise groups—whether they were walkers or marathon runners.

GETTING STARTED: TRAIN, DON'T STRAIN

If you have not exercised for months or years, begin slowly. If twenty minutes of walking puts a strain on your body, start with five or ten minutes instead. Twenty minutes is something you can build up to. But even in those five or ten minutes, you will begin to feel better and generate more NO.

You can toss out the "No pain, no gain" signs that you have been holding onto. Replace them with something like, "Train, don't strain." You do not need to exercise until it hurts, because even modest amounts of activity can protect you from serious illnesses and improve your chances of longevity. Your blood vessels will be healthier, and so will your heart.

It may have taken you many years to become as out of shape as you might be today. Give yourself time to get fit. Increase your workout a little at a time, and do not rush it. Begin by walking around the block if that feels most comfortable, and gradually add to your time and distance.

If you have physical limitations, do what you are capable of doing. Even if you walk with a cane, you can participate in some level of physical activity—perhaps just walking a hundred feet at a time. Try building some physical activity into your daily routine whenever possible—walking a few blocks to the supermarket is better than driving; climbing the stairs is better than using the elevator; walking the golf course pulling your clubs on wheels behind you or carrying them over your shoulder is healthier than using a cart. Even though sustained, aerobic activity in twenty or more minute increments is optimal, I am convinced that short bursts of NO-boosting exercise are also helpful to your overall well-being.

Gain Without Pain

"After four days on NO therapy, my sixty-four-year-old father was able to improve his running time by two minutes. I was able to start jogging and lifting weights again without any muscular soreness after having a baby."

Shelley, 29, Detroit

What Does Your Doctor Say About Exercise?

Most people can start the type of modest exercise program I recommend without any risks to their health. However, if you have led a sedentary lifestyle for years, contact your physician before you begin to work out. This is particularly important if you have a history of:

- Heart or vascular disease

- High blood pressure

- Chest pain

- Lung disease

- Joint problems (such as osteoarthritis)

- Fainting or dizzy spells

In some cases, your doctor may recommend that you undergo a treadmill test in which electrocardiogram readings are taken while you exercise. This test can detect any cardiovascular problems that might require some adjustments in your workout schedule. Keep in mind that virtually everyone—even those with heart disease—can incorporate some physical activity into his or her life. Talk with your doctor about the optimal exercise program for you.

SEEING RESULTS IN NO TIME

In the upcoming weeks and months, as you make physical activity a regular part of your life, you will begin to notice significant improvements in your capacity for exercise. Over time, your endothelial health will improve, and the accompanying increased production of NO will cause greater vasodilation and improved blood flow. That, in turn, will increase your ability to exercise. Your ten-minute workout will increase to twenty minutes, and then to thirty—and you will feel all the better for it.

To get even more out of your workout, try taking the recommended antioxidant supplements before exercising rather than at bedtime. It may improve your exercise capacity to take these supplements about thirty minutes before working out. During those thirty minutes, the antioxidants make their way into the bloodstream, and your endothelial cells begin generating more NO. You will often feel an extra boost of energy. There is a synergistic effect between exercise and the supplements, with your body producing more NO than it otherwise would. Most people will notice this kind of effect about three to four months after starting this regimen.

Down with the Blood Pressure, Up with the Stamina

Charlie, a forty-eight-year-old from Washington, D.C., has always been a physically active guy—devoted to running, lifting weights, and windsurfing. Despite all the exercise, he discovered that his blood pressure was at the border line of hypertension: 140/90. Then he heard about nitric oxide.

"When I first began the NO program," Charlie says, "my blood pressure immediately dropped thirty points, bringing me well within the optimal range. But it was in my athletic performance where the difference became most noticeable!

"I cut fifteen minutes off my old time for a five-mile run. The difference I feel going up hills is amazing. I hardly slow my pace at all. And I have a good 30 percent more stamina. It seems like I can just keep going forever without having to stop. My recovery has been improved dramatically too. The other day I did five hours of wind-surfing in a thirty-knot wind. Usually after a day like that I can barely walk for three days. With NO I woke up the next day and wasn't even sore."

With so much of athletic performance dependent upon the efficient flow of oxygen-rich blood to the muscles, it's not surprising that nitric oxide gives stamina a powerful boost.

Harvard Weighs in on Exercise and Life Span

A well-known study of nearly 17,000 Harvard male alumni examined a number of factors in their lifestyle that could contribute to their overall and cardiovascular well-being.

And clearly, exercise ended up at the head of the class. When the health of these men (ages thirty-five to seventy-four years) was evaluated, those who were less active had a 64 percent increased risk of a heart attack than their former classmates who were more active. Those who exercised also tended to live longer, with fewer deaths from all causes. The active men who expended 2,000 calories per week while exercising had mortality rates that were one fourth to one third lower than their sedentary contemporaries.

At this point, I am confident that you understand the critical importance of incorporating an exercise plan into your life. If you have not exercised in a long time, I understand that this portion of the **Say Yes to NO Plan** may seem impossible. If that thought is going through your mind, all I can tell you is that there is nothing more valuable to you than your health. You must take responsibility for your own life, and you have the opportunity right now to make one of the most important decisions of your life—and to commit to sticking with it. Many others have successfully accepted this challenge, and I know you can too.

What About Resistance Training Exercises?

I am mainly addressing exercise from the standpoint of boosting your nitric oxide production and reducing your risk of cardiovascular disease. My overwhelming message is that you do not need superstrenuous workout sessions or activities, but you do need to get your heart rate elevated for at least twenty minutes, three times a week. As you progress with your program, you will be capable of more—and most likely will want to do more.

While my recommendation is for aerobic exercise, it is also important to discuss resistance training. There is a rapidly growing body of research to show that resistance training is necessary to counter the muscle atrophy that accompanies aging. In order to prevent the loss of muscle mass as you age, you may want to include a resistance training component to your exercise regimen—once you have progressed to the level of aerobic fitness required to maintain my basic **Say Yes to NO** fitness plan.

Your resistance training should focus on a variety of eight to ten activities to work most of the major muscle groups. For each muscle group, you should perform one to three sets of eight to fifteen repetitions each. Keeping your major muscles active with even moderate resistance can provide significant benefits for muscle mass.

Lest you feel intimidated by the idea of having to lift weights, I want you to realize that you do not have to rely on equipment like barbells and dumbbells to do resistance training. You can get the same benefits from using inner tubes, elastics bands, hand weights, and wall pulleys. Just be sure that when you decide to start a resistance program, you do it at least twice a week—with proper form—to obtain the desired benefits. Think about it—three NO-boosting aerobic workouts and two resistance workouts a week. You and I both know you can work up to that level.

THE HEART OF THE MATTER

Before we move on, let's review what we have learned in this chapter.

- The acceleration of blood flow that occurs during exercise can stimulate the production of the enzyme NO synthase, which is important for the body's production of nitric oxide.

- Regular physical activity can reduce blood pressure and cholesterol levels.

- Exercise prevents blood platelets from adhering to vessel walls, lowering the likelihood of plaque accumulation and blood clotting.

- Make a commitment to integrate exercise into your life, at least twenty minutes a day, three or more days a week.

DR. IGNARRO'S SAY YES TO NO REGIMEN IN A NUTSHELL

The **Say Yes to NO** regimen is much more about lifestyle and mindset than it is about rigid guidelines. I do not give you meal plans or exercise routines. What I do want to convey is that your cardiovascular health comes down to making the right choices in three areas:

(1) NO-boosting supplements
(2) NO-boosting nutrition
(3) NO-boosting fitness

TIER 1: SAY YES TO NO-BOOSTING SUPPLEMENTS

CAUTION: Although I just said that my program is not about rigid guidelines, in the area of NO-boosting supplements, you must be uncompromising. You will only receive the full benefits if you follow the supplement program precisely as I suggest, because its effects are critically dependent upon the synergy between the prescribed amino acids and antioxidants. Beware of the potential confusion that can be caused by supplements on the market that claim to produce NO but which contain only L-arginine (usually in insufficient doses) and fail to take advantage of my discovery that it is the combination of nutrients that triggers cardiovascular health benefits. Do not be fooled—your health is too important.

Amino Acids

L-arginine and L-citrulline, the amino acids that stimulate your body's production of NO, are key ingredients of your supplement regimen. My recommended dosages are:

L-arginine: 4 to 6 grams (400 to 600 mg) per day, either taken all before bedtime or divided into morning and evening.

L-citrulline: 200 to 1,000 mg per day, taken along with the L-arginine.

Antioxidants

Antioxidants deactivate dangerous oxygen radicals in your body, helping to safeguard the health of your NO-producing endothelial cells. Here are my recommended doses of antioxidants (either synthesized or "natural"):

Vitamin C: 500 mg per day

Vitamin E: 200 IU per day (check with your doctor first if you take anticoagulants such as Coumadin or aspirin)

Folic acid: 400 to 800 mcg per day

Alpha lipoic acid: 10 mg per day

You can currently purchase each of these supplements on the Internet from:

www.LifeExtension.com
www.GNC.com
www.Savon.com
www.Drugstore.com

For more information on supplements, you may also visit my Web site at www.ignarrocom.

TIER 2: SAY YES TO NO-BOOSTING NUTRITION

NO-boosting nutrition is all about moderation, moderation, moderation—and a common sense lifestyle that involves controlling both your food choices and your portion sizes. Do not overdo it on any one food. Too much of a good thing can become a bad thing, but by all means avoid the bad and focus on the good!

Avoid Saturated Fats—They Increase Your "Bad" LDL Cholesterol

Avoid or cut back to minimal consumption of:

Fatty meats (beef, pork,
   lamb, veal, poultry skin)
Organ meats (liver)
Processed meats
   (hot dogs, salami)
Egg yolks

Cakes, cookies, and crackers
Pastry
White Bread
Butter and margarine
Potato chips
Taco chips

Dairy products (whole milk,	Buttered popcorn
cheese, cream cheese,	Fried potatoes
ice cream)	Commercial salad dressings

Say Yes to Heart-Friendly Fats

Any fat—bad or good—is high in calories and should be used sparingly. Here are the fats recommended by the American Heart Association:

Canola oil	Light and dark sesame oil
Corn oil	Vegetable oil
Safflower oil	Pure and virgin olive oil

Don't Forget Your Fiber

High intake of dietary fiber helps lower the rate of coronary artery disease. Gradually work your way up to 25 grams of fiber per day by eating:

Vegetables (raw or steamed)	Beans and peas
Fruit	Brown rice
Whole-grain breads	Bran
and cereals	Nuts and seeds

. . . and remember to drink at least 8 glasses of water a day!

Seafood—A Nutritional Windfall

The following seafoods are great sources of omega-3 fatty acids and NO-producing proteins:

Salmon   Snapper
Tuna   Swordfish
Mackerel   Lobster
Herring   Shrimp
Halibut   Cod
Sardines

Special Functional Foods to Keep You Heart-Healthy

Below is a list of foods with the uniquely powerful capacity to protect your cardiovascular health:

Egg whites   Dark chocolate
Garlic   Red wine
Green tea   Grape juice
Flaxseed   Blueberries
Soy   Pomegranate juice
Nuts

TIER 3: SAY YES TO NO-BOOSTING FITNESS

You do not have to become a fitness fanatic or a gym rat to make great improvements in your cardiovascular health through exercise. All I ask is that you do it in moderation (there is that word again). You will receive measurable benefits such as lower blood pressure and LDL cholesterol as well as the reduced risk of arterial plaque if you commit to at least twenty minutes of exercise, three times per week. More is even better, but I implore you to do at least this minimum amount. You can get these benefits from any of the following exercises:

Walking	Yoga
Jogging	Pilates
Bicycling	Cross-country skiing
Swimming	Jumping rope
Rowing	Rollerblading (in-line skating)
Tennis	Gardening
Squash	Dancing
Basketball	

. . . or anything else you find fun and will stick with!

The essence of my **Say Yes to NO** regimen is moderation, so do not go overboard with fitness—any more than you would with the other two elements of your healthy new lifestyle. Just remember: You must work your way up to a minimum of twenty minutes of exercise, at least three times per week.

9

NEW MIRACLES AROUND THE CORNER: THE NO BREAKTHROUGH SOARS INTO THE FUTURE

The more we learn about NO, the more impressive its curative powers become. In the foreseeable future, medicine will develop new healing techniques for even more major diseases based on the workings of nitric oxide.

In this book I have concentrated primarily on nitric oxide and cardiovascular disease. In this chapter, I will describe exciting developmental areas of NO research. Because of the miracle molecule, we may one day be capable of reducing the risk or severity of illnesses ranging from diabetes to rheumatoid arthritis, from cancer to Alzheimer's disease. The research findings are still preliminary with some of these conditions; in others the evidence is persuasive. The message is clear: If you can increase your levels of NO, you will be doing your body a favor in many ways, since virtually every organ and physiological process is dependent on nitric oxide.

With NO therapy you will be putting the brakes on cardiovascular disease, but you will also enjoy many other benefits. Here are some of them.

DIABETES AND THE NO FACTOR

If you are one of the 17 million Americans with diabetes, you already know how challenging this disease can be. Unless diabetes is carefully and effectively controlled, its complications can be dangerous and devastating. You have an increased likelihood of developing heart disease and high blood pressure. You are vulnerable to eye problems, called retinopathy, which can lead to blindness. You are prone to nerve damage or neuropathy. You are susceptible to kidney disease. Your hands, legs, and feet may bruise easily and heal slowly. You may even face circulatory problems in the lower limbs which could lead to amputation. Even if you are conscientiously following your doctor's recommendations regarding blood glucose measurements, medications, and diet, you are still not immune from serious complications. This is why nitric oxide is so important to diabetics.

NO Takes the Case

Despite the fact that there is no compelling evidence to date that NO can make insulin more available to the body, we do know it can intervene to help prevent potential complications. Most diabetic complications—from high blood pressure to eye problems to erectile dysfunction—are vascular in nature and are associated with high levels of oxidative stress that impair the endothelial cells. If you were to run tests on people with advanced diabetes, you would find that their endothelium is incapable of producing adequate amounts of NO. When that happens, diabetic complications almost always follow.

By implementing the strategies in this book, you can reduce

damage to your endothelial cells, boost your NO production, and halt the development and progression of diabetic complications. We know that nitric oxide can reduce blood pressure levels. We know that it plays a role in normal erectile function. We know that it can reduce the risk of diabetic retinopathy. Nitric oxide can make a great and positive difference in your quality of life.

"I Even Enjoy Walking"

"After being on NO therapy for three weeks, I noticed that my diabetic feet have feeling in them again and they aren't perpetually cold. The improvement seems to be a continuing thing. I even enjoy walking again!"

Judy, 58, Duluth

ERECTILE DYSFUNCTION AND THE NO FACTOR

Despite the tidal wave of Viagra jokes uttered by seemingly every comedian within reach of a microphone, erectile dysfunction is no laughing matter. Just ask the 15 to 30 million men who are chronically unable to attain or maintain an erection with sufficient rigidity for sexual intercourse. This disorder can damage self-esteem, lead to serious depression, and drive an emotional wedge between a man and his sexual partner.

For many years, men with erectile dysfunction were told that they suffered from a psychological dysfunction. Most physicians claimed "It's in your head," since they felt impotence stemmed from performance anxiety or sexual disinterest. We now know a lot more about erectile dysfunction, and medical science has changed its thinking. Physicians learned that the cause of impotence in most cases is physical, not psychological—and may often be a vascular problem.

When blood flow to the penis is constricted, there is no realistic chance for an erection, no matter how great the desire. My own research has shown that the erectile tissues of men with severe erectile dysfunction produce much less nitric oxide than men without this problem. Unless there is a way to increase their NO levels, erections simply are not going to be possible.

NO Takes the Case

Male sexual arousal is a complex process, but our research has demonstrated that NO can improve blood flow to the penis by stimulating the production of cyclic GMP directly in the erectile tissue. High levels of NO can raise cyclic GMP concentrations by a startling one hundred times. As blood flow increases and erectile tissue dilates, an erection is produced.

If you look at the demographics of impotence, you will see that men are more likely to develop this condition as they age. According to the Endocrine Society, erectile dysfunction is a chronic problem in 10 percent of men in their sixties, 25 percent in their seventies, and 40 percent in their eighties. There is a parallel decline of NO levels in elderly men. Many of the diseases that have a NO connection—not only erectile dysfunction, but also high blood pressure, atherosclerosis, urinary incontinence, diabetes, and perhaps Alzheimer's disease—are much more common in older individuals, coinciding with apparent decreases in NO production.

What a Perk

"I am a thirty-four-year-old male and suffer from minor erectile dysfunction. I started NO therapy as protection against heart disease. Then I noticed that my sex life was improving. About three weeks after starting to boost my NO, my erectile function began to improve until it was normal after about four months. What an amazing health breakthrough when you can rise to the occasion and protect your heart at the same time."

                                        Jerry, 34, Atlantic City

---

Since Viagra's introduction in 1998, you could not have read a newspaper or watched TV without understanding that the drug has revolutionized the treatment of erectile dysfunction. This blue pill works through a mechanism that has evolved from NO research. Viagra increases the dilating activity of cyclic GMP, which results in erections.

Though the diet, supplements, and exercise program in this book will strengthen your endothelium and increase your NO production, there is not yet any proof that NO alone will resolve erectile dysfunction. If this is a problem that affects you, you must consult your doctor.

RHEUMATOID ARTHRITIS AND THE NO FACTOR

For about two million Americans, rheumatoid arthritis is an unwelcome and, in some cases, a crippling part of their day-to-day existence. Imagine the small joints in your hands aching so badly that you can barely grip a bottle of pain-killing medication that might provide some temporary escape from the debilitating discomfort. Or picture the joints in your wrists, knuckles, and feet so swollen, so red, and so deformed that they are almost too tender to touch. That is what living with rheumatoid arthritis is often like.

Rheumatoid arthritis is an inflammatory disorder, believed to occur when the body's immune system attacks the synovial membrane that lines the joints. An acute inflammatory response within the body is frequently a positive and protective mechanism. The body's natural defense against invading microorganisms, triggering swelling as white blood cells attack and engulf the problematic bacteria, viruses, or parasites. But inflammation can be a double-edged sword. It can go to extremes and actually start destroying the tissue it was intended to defend. Over time, the synovium can thicken and damage the tendons, ligaments, cartilage, and bone. The resulting condition is rheumatoid arthritis.

"My Arthritis Pain Has Essentially Disappeared!"

"I suffer from rheumatoid arthritis and I experience joint stiffness and leg and hand pain every morning on awakening. About one month after commencing nitric oxide therapy, I noticed a dramatic improvement in my condition. That is, my joints were not as stiff as before and, even more dramatically, the pains in my hands and legs essentially disappeared. I have never experienced better effects with any prescription drug."

Alice, 54, London, England

NO Takes the Case

Nitric oxide could produce a reversal of fortune for rheumatoid arthritis sufferers, blocking exaggerated inflammatory processes by means of a number of mechanisms:

- NO is a potent antioxidant and also an anti-inflammatory. It can minimize oxidative stress and its effects within the body, including inflammation, and thus can help minimize the effects of rheumatic arthritis.
- NO can interact with enzymes and genes that play a role in inflammation. As it turns off these enzymes, it can reduce the severity of the inflammation.
- NO relaxes the blood vessels, which promotes blood flow and healing.

Most people's bodies are well equipped to produce greater amounts of NO when threatened by inflammation. The enzyme called NO synthase, which stimulates the synthesis of NO, is produced in greater amounts during inflammation and infection. As NO levels rise, the body can more effectively combat the rheumatoid arthritis-related inflammation.

One other point about rheumatoid arthritis must be mentioned: Some rheumatoid arthritis sufferers are confused over research suggesting that there may be a large overproduction of NO in the inflamed joints themselves—which may produce a worsening of joint destruction. Others believe that the overproduction of NO actually serves a protective function. Research to date has shown that the supplements I recommend do not increase NO production in the joints. These supplements increase the levels of NO only in the endothelial cells of the blood vessels. The likelihood is you will be combating the inflammatory process, not facilitating it.

CANCER AND THE NO FACTOR

This year alone, more than one million Americans will be diagnosed with cancer. In an instant, their lives will be transformed as they gear up to fight this fearful disease. Thanks to continuing medical advances, more cancer patients will survive than succumb. Even so, the path to healing can be an enormous physical, emotional, and spiritual challenge.

As you may already know, cancer proliferates according to a complex process called *carcinogenesis*. Initially, one or more genes are damaged, causing mutations that produce abnormal cells which can begin to grow rapidly and without restraint. These deviant cells can proliferate for years, attaching themselves to other aberrant cells before they finally become detectable, either by means of screening tests or after symptoms appear. The earlier these tumors or masses of cancer cells are detected, the better the prognosis.

NO Takes the Case

Nitric oxide appears to be one of our most powerful allies as the body mobilizes for war against this life-threatening cellular disorder. NO can inhibit the growth of cancer cells—not only in the earliest stages when there may be only a few undetected cells, but also later in the disease process. High levels of NO may be able to slow cancer cell proliferation, keeping the cancer in a holding pattern long enough for the body's own immune system to prepare to destroy malignant cells on its own. Some researchers have theorized that one of the most important functions of NO is to prevent the onset of various cancers by inhibiting abnormal cell growth.

Evidence of NO as a cancer inhibitor is now well documented. A chronic surge of oxidative stress appears to play a key role in the promotion of cancer, perhaps because of the damage to DNA caused by free radicals. As a powerful antioxidant, NO can derail the growth of abnormal cells involved in many types of cancers and keep the cancer at bay. My own laboratory conducted a study (published in the *American Journal of Physiology* in 1997) demonstrating that NO can inhibit the growth of human colon cancer cells. We could even describe the mechanism involved. Less certain is whether NO can prevent the development of cancer altogether.

A number of studies have shown that you may be able to reduce your cancer risk by simply increasing your intake of antioxidants in the diet and supplements, which are an important component of the supplement package I suggest.

The Efficacy of Nutrients in the Fight Against Cancer

At the University of Helsinki in Finland, more than 29,000 male smokers (ages fifty to sixty-nine) received supplements of either alpha-tocopherol (vitamin E, 50 mg), beta-carotene (20 mg), both of these nutrients, or a placebo. In a report published in the *Journal of the National Cancer Institute* in 1998, after a median follow-up of 6.1 years, those taking alpha-tocopherol

showed a 32 percent decline in their incidence of prostate cancer, compared with those not receiving this supplement; mortality from prostate cancer was 41 percent lower in this vitamin
group. (By contrast, individuals taking only beta-carotene actually had a higher incidence of prostate cancer.)

We can now say that the future of NO-based cancer therapy
looks quite promising. A number of pharmaceutical companies
are working to develop new drugs that would target tumor sites
within the body, and bathe the area in NO in order to block the
growth and metastasis or spread of certain solid tumors and
leukemias.

ULCERS AND THE NO FACTOR

Gastric ulcers are actually irritations of the membrane that lines
the stomach and the duodenum, the upper small intestine. If
you have ever had an ulcer, you know all too well that it can
cause excruciating pain, most often in the hours after eating,
along with nausea, vomiting, and precipitous weight loss.

For many years, doctors thought the cause of ulcers was
stress and advised patients to reduce the tension in their lives,
switch to a bland diet, and drink lots of milk to coat the stomach. Researchers have since discovered that a particular type of
bacterium—called *Helicobacter pylori* (or *H. pylori*)—can thrive in
the digestive tract and may well cause a weakening in the protective lining of the stomach and duodenum. Consequently,
most ulcers are treated with antibiotics.

NO Takes the Case

While bacterial infection clearly appears to be a factor in the development of gastric ulcers, it is not the only one. A growing body of evidence strongly suggests that impairment of blood flow in the vessels and the mucosal lining of the stomach and duodenum contribute to the ulcerative process. When blood flow in the region declines, even modestly, irritations leading to ulcerations are more likely to develop. If you suffer from ulcers and begin adopting strategies to restore normal blood flow—including those that elevate NO levels—you may be able to reduce substantially the severity of your symptoms.

Here is something else to keep in mind about ulcers. Medical researchers recognize that long-term use of certain medications—most notably such anti-inflammatory drugs as aspirin, ibuprofen, and naproxen—can interfere with the formation of prostaglandins—hormonelike substances that help control blood pressure, muscle contractions, and inflammation. Although the prostaglandins serve beneficial purposes within the body, their production of pain and inflammation while combating injuries can be uncomfortable—hence the use of anti-inflammatories to block their action.

Unfortunately, another essential activity of prostaglandins that gets blocked by the blanket effect of anti-inflammatories is the dilation of blood vessels to maintain normal blood flow in the gastrointestinal tract. The result is an increased vulnerability of the stomach to ulcerations. Fortunately, a high level of NO can overcome this effect, keeping blood flowing regularly and preventing ulcerations. If you maintain high NO levels, you should be able to take anti-inflammatories without running the risk of developing ulcers.

Vasodilation is crucial to maintaining the health of the gastrointestinal tract. At least one pharmaceutical company is presently conducting research that suggests that when NO is delivered to the gastric mucous membrane, it can not only prevent but actually heal ulcers—100 percent of them—simply by restoring normal blood flow to the stomach and intestinal lining.

URINARY INCONTINENCE AND THE NO FACTOR

As we age beyond fifty, we become increasingly susceptible to uncontrollable and involuntary loss of urine, termed urinary incontinence. Loss of bladder control affects approximately thirteen million adults in the United States, affecting twice as many women as men. Urinary incontinence too often creates anxiety and encourages social isolation. Many people with this problem are too embarrassed to discuss the problem even with their doctor.

Researchers have identified a number of causes of incontinence, including urinary tract infections and an array of different medications, most notably diuretics, sedatives, narcotics, antihistamines, antidepressants, and calcium channel blockers. There is also evidence that, in many cases, the bladder simply cannot properly relax. Even when the bladder is only partially full, the urge to urinate cannot be suppressed, with leakage increasing due to a sneeze, cough, or laugh.

NO Takes the Case

Medical science has learned that deficiencies in nitric oxide production are unquestionably a factor in incontinence. Under normal circumstances, NO does an excellent job of relaxing the bladder's smooth muscle, permitting it to expand normally and fill with urine. When deficiencies do occur, the bladder cannot relax sufficiently and releases some of its urine—either involuntarily or with abnormal frequency.

By boosting your levels of NO, you may be able to reduce or eliminate incontinence. Some pharmaceutical companies are investigating the feasibility of developing new drugs that stimulate the production of NO specifically in the nerves leading to the bladder wall, causing dilation and relaxation that may well restore normal bladder functioning.

Although more is known about the association between NO and urinary incontinence in women, this problem plagues both sexes. Most urologists believe that the underlying cause of incontinence is similar in men and women, and the approaches to managing the problem may be the same as well. Further research on the benefits of NO are underway.

ALZHEIMER'S DISEASE AND THE NO FACTOR

This terrifying and devastating brain disorder already affects more than four million elderly Americans, impairing their memory, language, and reasoning ability. The number of afflicted is expected to rise as the population ages.

Although there are still many unanswered questions about Alzheimer's, our understanding of it is increasing exponentially. We know, for example, that the brains of Alzheimer's sufferers have high levels of abnormal structures called beta-amyloid plaques, which are deposits of protein and cellular material. Some researchers believe that these plaques directly cause Alzheimer's; others hypothesize that they may be a byproduct or marker of the brain changes that occur with the illness, including the progressive destruction of brain neurons. Some research shows that as NO levels decline in these patients, there is a marked acceleration of the formation of these plaques.

NO Takes the Case

Studies also indicate that the beta-amyloid plaques accumulate in response to increases in oxidative stress in the brain. A key strategy for reducing the risk of Alzheimer's disease may be to increase the body's production of NO and to consume higher levels of vitamins E, C, and other antioxidants. A number of recent studies have examined the effects of vitamin intake on the risk of Alzheimer's disease:

Can Vitamin E Slow the Progress of Alzheimer's?

In an Alzheimer's Disease Cooperative Study, researchers evaluated the influence of vitamin E (alpha-tocopherol) on the progression of Alzheimer's disease in more than 300 men and women whose disorder was moderately severe. A report published in the *New England Journal of Medicine* in 1997 described one group of individuals who took 2000 IU of vitamin E a day for two years, while two other groups took either another supplement (selegiline, 10 mg a day) or a placebo.

Investigators monitored a number of parameters in these patients, including the time elapsed until the loss of the ability to dress, bathe, and use the toilet independently; the development of severe dementia (total disorientation, hallucinations); the need for institutionalization; and death. After two years, the men and women taking vitamin E fared better than the other two groups with a slowing of the progression of their disease. The vitamin E group reached the disease endpoints 230 days later than those taking the placebo.

Some scientists believe that NO is intimately involved in the preservation and enhancement of learning and memory. They are convinced that a deficiency in NO could be at least one cause of Alzheimer's disease. Much more research is needed. A current area of investigation is aimed at developing pharmaceutical agents that can stimulate NO production in targeted regions of the brain in the hope that it will decrease the quantity of beta-amyloid plaques.

Folic Acid's Impact on Brain Health

At the National Institute on Aging, scientists conducted an animal study, using mice with Alzheimer's-like plaques in their brains. One group of these mice was fed a diet with normal amounts of folic acid, while a second group consumed a folic acid-deficient diet. In the *Journal of Neuroscience* in 2002, the researchers described how they counted neurons in the hippocampus region of the brains of mice at the end of the study. They found that those mice fed the folic acid-rich diet had a greater number of neurons than those on the deficiency diet.

When you take the antioxidant supplements described in this book, I believe you may be lowering your risk of developing Alzheimer's disease, possibly by reducing oxidative stress, and promoting NO production.

NO AND OTHER DISEASES

In addition to the link between nitric oxide deficiencies and rheumatoid arthritis, low levels of NO also may be associated with other inflammatory diseases, including Crohn's disease and irritable bowel syndrome. Some researchers believe that Crohn's disease, an inflammatory bowel disorder, may be caused by an NO imbalance. That is, patients with Crohn's disease may experience waves of increasing and decreasing NO production.

Studies have examined a possible role of NO deficiencies in multiple sclerosis. According to one hypothesis, deficits in NO may contribute to the exacerbation of multiple sclerosis, and higher levels of NO may ease disease symptoms. There is another school of thought that byproducts of the interaction between NO and free radicals may actually worsen multiple sclerosis. The research to date is very preliminary, and it is much too early to conclude definitively whether NO plays any role in multiple sclerosis.

ONLY THE BEGINNING

As research progresses, NO appears more and more to be a multipurpose disease fighter: NO seems to play a necessary role in fighting infections. Research has shown that when an infectious organism invades the body, a component of that organism triggers the production of large amounts of NO synthase, which is the enzyme needed for the production of NO. In turn, NO seems to be the single most important molecule in white blood cells, which are on the leading edge of the body's defense against disease. Thus, NO appears to be a key player in destroying or interfering with the growth of these invading organisms.

A CLOSING THOUGHT

When I think that I played a role in discovering a tiny molecule with the potential to eradicate so many of mankind's scourges, I feel very proud, very humble—and very fortunate. Scientific research should not be conducted in a vacuum, but rather with an eye toward its ultimate value to society. If the work described in this book, to which I have dedicated my life, can help you and your loved ones to live longer, healthier lives, then I will have received my greatest reward

THE HEART OF THE MATTER

Before we move on, let's review what you have learned in this chapter.

NO research is ongoing in a number of areas, showing promise in fields in addition to cardiovascular disease. People with (or at risk for) the following conditions are already benefiting, or might soon be helped, by the ongoing studies of NO:

- Diabetes
- Erectile dysfunction
- Rheumatoid arthritis
- Cancer

- Ulcers
- Urinary incontinence
- Alzheimer's disease
- Infections
- Inflammatory diseases (e.g., Crohn's disease)
- Multiple sclerosis

10

NITRIC OXIDE: SOME FINAL THOUGHTS

One out of every two Americans will die from cardiovascular disease—which in almost every case could have been prevented. I wrote this book to help you do just that.

ADVANCES IN CARDIOVASCULAR MEDICINE

We live in a time of astounding medical advances that provide today's cardiologists with more tools than doctors a generation ago could even have imagined. Techniques and treatments that were unknown until recently—from angioplasty to magnetic resonance imaging, from tissue plasminogen activators to drug-eluting stents—are indicative of the strides made by medical researchers.

At the same time, more medications are available to combat disorders like high blood pressure and high cholesterol than ever before. For example, diuretics and beta-blockers were once the only drugs available to physicians for treating hypertension, but today your doctor can choose from among calcium-channel blockers, ACE inhibitors, angiotensin II receptor blockers, and alpha-adrenergic receptor blockers.

Though these medications have saved many lives by reducing blood pressure readings to safer levels, they are expensive and can cause such serious side effects as stomach problems, dizziness, insomnia, rash, and swelling. No wonder many people have simply stopped taking them. No wonder they are willing to put themselves at risk rather than continue using them.

I think we all know deep down that for long term health, there has to be another way—one that works more closely in unison with our bodies. Whether you are already taking prescription drugs, or worry that you might have to someday, maximizing your body's production of nitric oxide is a natural alternative that may make hypertension medication unnecessary. Unlike prescription medications, NO therapy is inexpensive and has no side effects.

GO WITH NO

As you have learned, one of your most powerful allies in maintaining your heart health is this remarkable molecule called NO, which was once overlooked as little more than an ozone-destroying pollutant. Today, we have strong evidence that NO is a very strong protector of the cardiovascular system.

Though it is manufactured in the body in only minute amounts and is quite unstable, nitric oxide can cause life-saving relaxation of your arteries and veins. Its biological activity can reduce blood pressure and positively influence every other component of the cardiovascular system, while at the same time affecting the brain, the lungs, the gastrointestinal system, the immune system, sexual function, the peripheral nerves, and nearly every other organ and process in the human body.

Persuasive as the evidence has become in recent years, I am convinced that NO research is only in its infancy. When I won the Nobel Prize for my discoveries in this field, I knew that what we had already learned about nitric oxide was significant, but it was just scratching the surface. Many other scientists agreed, and they are now turning their attention to NO as well.

When I edited a textbook, *Nitric Oxide: Biology and Pathobiology,* published in 2000, researchers from around the globe contributed to it. Chapters were written not only by American scientists at such institutions as Harvard Medical School, Duke University, Stanford University, the Mayo Clinic, Johns Hopkins University, UCLA, Yale University, Cornell University, Emory University, and the National Cancer Institute, but also by investigators from Canada, the United Kingdom, Germany, France, Belgium, Sweden, Uruguay, Argentina, Turkey, and Japan. When we write the second edition of this text, I am convinced that the level of participation will broaden even further.

More and more research dollars—allocated by the National Institutes of Health as well as many other funding sources—are now supporting NO studies. They are focused not only on how NO may help prevent or resolve a host of major diseases, but also on achieving a better understanding of nitric oxide's basic biology and chemistry.

Due to the rapid pace of this research, there is a now a virtual deluge of scientific articles being submitted to *Nitric Oxide,* the professional journal I founded, and to other scientific publications, including the most prestigious in the field, among them the *Proceedings of the National Academy of Sciences.*

At the same time, pharmaceutical companies are actively developing drugs that will leverage the power of NO to reduce the risk of high blood pressure, atherosclerosis, strokes, ulcers, urinary incontinence, Alzheimer's disease, and inflammatory disorders. Early reports about these compounds are extremely encouraging. Imagine a medication, for instance, in which nitric oxide molecules are combined with aspirin or ibuprofen. Once the NO is released in the stomach, it will prevent the development of gastric irritation and ulcers so often associated with anti-inflammatory and pain-relieving medications. These NO-based medications appear safe, and I expect them to become available—first as prescription drugs and subsequently over-the-counter—in the near future.

The years ahead will be exciting times for those of us involved with the curative potential of NO—and most importantly, for people like you who will benefit from it.

HEART PRESERVERS: THE NEXT GENERATION

There are heart-healthy nutrients on the horizon that when synergized will add even more potency to your NO production. While research continues, I would like to mention a few nutrients I believe hold the brightest promise.

Coenzyme Q10

Although this powerful antioxidant has been available as a supplement for years in Europe and Japan, it is only now being considered a breakthrough in the treatment of cardiovascular disease by American scientists.

Coenzyme Q10 (CoQ10) is a fat-soluble molecule that performs several major bodily functions, among them disarming free radicals. The "Q" in coenzyme Q10 stands for *quinone,* a molecule with similarities to vitamin E. The "10" refers to the molecule's ten units of carbon atoms.

All of us produce some of our own CoQ10, and it is actually found in every cell in the body. It must be present to produce ATP, the energy manufactured within the cells that keeps us going. If your CoQ10 levels are deficient, you are likely to feel run down and burned out.

CoQ10 and NO As a particularly effective antioxidant, CoQ10 interacts with enzymes already in the body to trigger the chemical reactions that inactivate free radicals, converting them into safe substances before LDL cholesterol can be oxidized. At the same time, it stimulates the activity of other antioxidants in the body, including vitamin E, working synergistically to keep these antioxidants in an active form and regenerating or "recycling" them even in the presence of free radicals, thus protecting the endothelial cells and insuring the body's ability to produce NO.

The body does not make enough CoQ10 to maximize its physiological benefits. We do consume CoQ10 in such functional foods as salmon, nuts, and such organ meats as liver, but probably not all that we need. Since CoQ10 production declines as we age, researchers believe low levels of the antioxidant contribute to age-related diseases, ranging from cardiovascular problems to cancer.

Heartening News About Coenzyme Q10

Clinical studies show that deficiency in CoQ10 is common in about 75 percent of cardiac patients. Because the heart is so metabolically active and needs a constant supply of fuel for contraction, it is unusually susceptible to CoQ10 deficiencies. Research points to the use of CoQ10 as a supplement for the treatment of such heart problems as:

- Angina pectoris (heart pain)

- Congestive heart failure (impairment of the heart to pump enough blood)

- Cardiac arrhythmias (irregular heartbeat)

- Cardiomyopathy (impairment of the heart muscle)

- Hyperthyroid heart failure

- Mitral valve prolapse

- High blood pressure

Weighing the Evidence

Studies have demonstrated that coenzyme Q10 can decrease blood pressure readings and reduce the risk and severity of congestive heart failure. For example:

- At the Institute of Biomedical Research at the University of Texas in Austin, 109 patients with hypertension were placed on high doses of coenzyme Q10 (varying from 75 to 360 mg a day) for four months. As the researchers reported in *Molecular Aspects of Medicine* in 1994, systolic blood pressure readings showed a mean decline from 159 to 147 mm Hg, while diastolic pressure decreased from 94 to 85 mm Hg. Remarkably, because of these improvements in blood pressure levels, 51 percent of the patients were able to discontinue from one to three of their blood pressure medications at an average of 4.4 months after they began taking coenzyme Q10—including a 40 percent decrease in the use of diuretics, a 59 percent drop in beta blockers, a 32 percent decline in ACE inhibitors, and a 28 percent decrease in calcium channel blockers. No side effects were seen with CoQ10 use.

- Italian researchers who were members of the CoQ10 Drug Surveillance Investigators Team studied 2,664 patients with congestive heart failure (CHF), using coenzyme Q10 as an adjunctive treatment. The daily dosage ranged from 50 to 150 mg, with most patients taking 100 mg a day. After three months, 54 percent of the patients showed improvements in at least three of their CHF symptoms, indicating a better quality of life. For example, as reported in *The Clinical Investigator* in 1993, 75 percent of the patients experienced a decrease in heart palpitations, 80 percent noted a decline in sweating, 49 percent had a decrease in liver enlargement, and 63 percent showed a decrease in subjective arrhythmias.

My hope is that in the next few years, science will develop a CoQ10 supplement of sufficient strength to help prevent—and even reverse—the cardiovascular damage done by aging and disease.

Krill Oil

Krill oil is a substance extracted from a shrimplike crustacean found in the waters of Antarctica. It is a cardiovascular home run, featuring a synergistic combination of phospholipids, life-essential membrane nutrients, omega-3 fatty acids, and such antioxidants as vitamins A and E.

In human studies, krill oil supplementation has been shown to support the heart and sugar levels, energy production, athletic performance, and healthy joints, as well as lowering LDL cholesterol and easing PMS symptoms. Krill oil is unique in featuring phospholipids specially integrated with omega-3 essential fatty acids and antioxidants. This desirable synergy works tirelessly to prevent cellular irritation and cardiovascular imbalance.

Krill Oil and NO Krill oil's antioxidant properties are three hundred times those of vitamins A and E and forty-eight times those of most fish oils. Plus the fact that the essential fatty acids of omega-3s are the building blocks for the phospholipids, which in turn are the building blocks for your cell membranes—the protective layer and gatekeeper of your cells. As the result of its potent synergy, krill oil works hard to keep the endothelium in good repair by deactivating free radicals, enabling optimal NO production.

Weighing the Evidence

Long-term krill oil safety was evaluated in a six-month study using mice as subjects. The mice were fed krill oil in a dosage which for humans would be 23.1 grams (for a 150-pound person), or seven to eleven times the recommended dose. No adverse effects or pathological findings were reported in any of the organ systems.

With such incredible cardiovascular benefits, krill oil is destined to become part of everybody's daily supplement package in the near future.

L-Taurine

You may not have heard of this amino acid, but I can assure you that you will soon be hearing a lot about it.

L-taurine is a semi-essential amino acid compound and a component of bile acids, which the body uses to help absorb fats and fat-soluble vitamins. It is also an antioxidant and in that role helps regulate the heartbeat and maintain cell membrane stability. L-taurine is found in such foods as eggs, dairy products, meats, and fish proteins. Since these foods, with the exception of fish, tend to be high in saturated fats, your best bet for L-taurine is to take it in nutraceutical form as a supplement.

L-taurine and NO L-taurine comprises over 50 percent of the total free amino acids in the heart. It has a positive effect on cardiac tissue and has been shown in some studies not only to lower blood pressure but also to strengthen the heart muscle, stabilize heart rhythm, and prevent blood clotting.

L-taurine is also an antioxidant that chases down free radicals, thereby protecting NO and maintaining stability in the endothelial membranes.

Weighing the Evidence

Many studies have been done to test the efficacy of L-taurine. Here are several examples:

- At the University of Shizuoka in Japan, researchers demonstrated that L-taurine can decrease LDL ("bad") cholesterol while increasing HDL ("good") cholesterol. The study was done by feeding a high cholesterol diet to rats for two weeks. Half the rats were also given L-taurine supplements and half were not. After two weeks, the serum cholesterol readings of the two groups showed that, compared to the group without supplementation, the L-taurine group had effectively been able to combat the harmful effects of the high cholesterol diet on LDL and HDL levels.

- Another Japanese study concluded that L-taurine effectively improves metabolism in rats. By looking at two groups of rats—L-taurine and placebo—the researchers found that insulin resistance and abdominal fat accumulations were significantly lower in the L-taurine–supplemented group. Concentrations of LDL cholesterol were also significantly lower in the L-taurine–supplemented group. In a complex chain of reasoning, the researchers deduced that L-taurine increased nitric oxide production, which in turn caused a decrease in cholesterol, which then led to an enhanced metabolism.

- In a study done by the Medical College of Georgia in Augusta, the effects of L-taurine depletion on blood vessel relaxation response were studied in rats. The researchers found that L-taurine depletion increases the ability of smooth muscle tissue to contract, but it decreases the muscle's ability to relax. Their findings also noted that depletion of L-taurine leads to impaired endothelium-dependent response, which is associated with reduced nitric oxide production, contributing to a decrease in vasorelaxant responses. "In plain English," the researchers concluded, "this simply means that depletion in L-taurine leads to reduced nitric oxide production leading to more tension in the walls of the blood vessels." Tension in the blood vessels impairs normal blood flow and can cause premature aging, disability, memory impairment, and dementia.

Because sufficient levels of L-taurine have been found to prevent brain overactivity and reduce platelet aggregation in diabetic patients, this substance may someday play a major role in controlling or preventing diabetes, and even Alzheimer's disease.

Selenium

This antioxidant is so remarkably effective that I predict it will be an integral synergizing element in the next generation of cardiovascular-friendly multivitamin supplements.

Selenium is an essential trace mineral in the human body, which can be derived from plants, and is essential to normal functioning of the immune system and thyroid gland. The full range of its antioxidant powers is only now being studied, but we do know that—in addition to its heart-healthy duties—selenium seems to reduce the inflammation of rheumatoid arthritis and may play a curative role in some forms of cancers.

Selenium and NO Selenium is an important part of the group of antioxidant enzymes that protect cells against the effects of free radicals produced during normal oxygen metabolism. By heading off these unstable molecules, selenium ensures that the endothelial cells will be free to produce maximal nitric oxide, resulting in greatly improved cardiovascular health.

Weighing the Evidence

In 2002, the *Doctor Yourself* newsletter reported: "Selenium has been shown to be protective against heart disease by animal studies, epidemiological studies, lab animal studies, and human studies. Selenium helps in maintaining the integrity of heart and artery tissue, regulation of blood pressure, regulation of blood clotting, and the reduction of plaque, or cholesterol, deposits in arteries."

Selenium is sure to play a major role in the future of cardiovascular health.

Silicon

In the human body, silicon is a trace mineral found in the highest concentrations in connective tissue such as blood vessels, cartilage, tendons, bone, collagen, and skin. Silicon is helpful in keeping blood vessel walls healthy (the aorta is especially rich in silicon), and it has been found that silicon levels decrease in arterial vessels with increasing age and the onset of atherosclerosis.

Silicon and NO Research indicates that silicon plays an important role in the health of our arteries by assuring the integrity of elastic fibers in the blood vessel wall. This elasticity helps to make the artery wall impermeable to the fatty infiltration and calcium deposition associated with plaque formation.

Just as antioxidants provide protection for NO and its production in the endothelium, silicon supports the underlying physical structure of the endothelium and blood vessel wall. Ongoing research on silicon and its relationship to NO and vascular health makes it an important nutrient in the scope of our developing understanding of cardiovascular nutrition.

Phytosterols

Science is just beginning to discover the ability of plant cholesterols to lower human LDL serum cholesterol. It works especially well when synergized with vitamin E.

Plant phytosterols, which are found in rice bran, wheat germ, corn oils, and soybeans, are compounds with chemical structures similar to that of animal cholesterol. Phytosterols, unlike cholesterol derived from animal sources—which raises the body's own cholesterol levels—are present only at very low levels in the body, because they are difficult to absorb. Phytosterols can actually block food-based LDL serum cholesterol from being absorbed into the blood stream. As you begin to digest your supper, these plant cholesterols take over the LDL serum cholesterols, causing less to be absorbed by your body. Consequently, both plant cholesterol and LDL serum cholesterol are excreted in waste matter.

Phytosterols and NO By substantially lowering LDL serum cholesterol, phytosterols help maintain cellular stability, giving the endothelial cells a healthy climate in which to produce nitric oxide, which in turn keeps the vessels relaxed and clean.

Weighing the Evidence

Science is quite aware of phytosterols' ability to block absorption of LDL serum cholesterol. We are now discovering that they may reduce an enlarged prostate, improve the blood sugar level of diabetics, and reduce inflammation in people with rheumatoid arthritis. Studies have shown that phytosterols taken daily in foods or in supplements can lower LDL serum cholesterol by an average of 10 to 14 percent. On account of these strong findings, in 2001 the National Cholesterol Panel issued a recommendation that plant cholesterol be incorporated into any cholesterol-lowering regimen.

Any day now, the substances you have just read about will be available in mega-cardiovascular multivitamins—compounds which will introduce you to a brave new world of cardiovascular health.

THE CARDIOVASCULAR RENAISSANCE

Medicine is on the brink of rethinking the protocols for treating heart disease—largely on the basis of nitric oxide. Even so, ask the average man on the street to tell you what he knows about nitric oxide, and he will probably still think of laughing gas, if anything comes to mind at all. That is beginning to change—as I can tell you from personal experience.

Before long, I expect nitric oxide to be a term as universally understood as cholesterol. I believe this book will help make a difference in accelerating the public's understanding of the importance of NO to its own well-being.

A New Life

James, a sixty-year-old retired fire chief from Oregon, spent sixteen years in the trenches, and it took its toll. Having to be on call 24/7, James could expect to be summoned for duty in the middle of the night, which meant he had to come fully awake in seconds. Even after he left the department, he retained this hypervigilance and was incapable of sleeping deeply through the night. To make matters worse, when he did manage to nod off, James was plagued by nightmares in which he relived the horrors and tragedies he had witnessed on the job. Ultimately, he was diagnosed with post-traumatic stress disorder.

In 1981, in addition to his psychological difficulties, James developed life-threatening physical problems—including high blood pressure, almost certainly abetted by the post-traumatic stress, difficulty breathing because the bottom third of his lungs were full of fluid, frequent bouts of pneumonia, even peritonitis. His doctors told him his cardiovascular distress was caused by the smoke he had inhaled on a daily basis for more than a decade and recommended he sue the state of Oregon for damages. The judge ruled in his favor and ordered the state to pay all James's medical bills for the rest of his life.

James, who had always been a physically active man, was a very depressed, semi-invalid from 1980 to 2003. Then, in May of 2003, he heard about nitric oxide therapy, which was said to offer hope to people in his condition. Almost immediately after starting NO therapy, he was, in his words, "sleeping like a rock." Three days after James began taking my recommended supplement regimen including amino acids and antioxidants, his blood pressure dropped from 170/90 to 164/80. When his lungs were tested in June of that year, they were clear. They were 100 percent clear in July and again in November. Last April, James did have pneumonia, but it was not severe enough to require oxygen or a prolonged recovery period. "I can breathe right down to my toes!" he exclaims.

Best of all, James has surged back into the world full-strength with more energy than he had before he got sick. He publishes a scuba diving magazine, enjoys work as a carpenter, even climbs roofs that need repair. NO therapy gave James a new life. For him, nitric oxide is literally "the miracle molecule."

THE NO MOMENT IS NOW

You do not have to wait for the rest of the world to see the light—and the drug companies to put new NO-based prescription drugs on the market—in order to take advantage of much of what NO has to offer. The supplements, the dietary recommendations and the exercise guidelines that I have described in this book are simple, safe, and effective ways to reduce the oxidative stress in your body, protect your endothelial cells, and maximize your production of NO, resulting in better health and a lower risk of heart ailments and other chronic diseases.

We have all made mistakes in the way we have lived our lives in the past. Maybe you have not exercised in years. Maybe you used to be a heavy smoker. Maybe you still are. Maybe you have consistently eaten meals with too much dietary fat and too few vegetables and fruits. Lucky for you, the body will be very forgiving once you put yourself on the right track.

You now have information mapped out for you on what you should be eating, the supplements you should be taking, and the active lifestyle you should be leading. Beginning today, you can turn your health and well-being around.

In these closing pages, let's briefly review the key elements of the program that I have recommended.

JUST DO IT

If you have heart disease or high blood pressure, the information in this book may change your life. You have probably read things in *NO More Heart Disease* that your doctor has never brought up—perhaps because he is not yet fully familiar with the breadth of NO research. Though the drug prescriptions he writes certainly have value—and you certainly should never stop taking them without his approval any more than you should start any new health regimen without consulting him—wouldn't you prefer to adopt safe, effective, and less expensive approaches rather than taking powerful chemicals with all of their potential side effects to manage your cardiovascular symptoms?

Even if you do not show signs of developing cardiovascular problems, simply reading this book while lying on the couch will not do a thing to safeguard your cardiovascular future. There is no such thing as a free lunch. If your goal is optimal health, make a commitment to spend a few minutes exercising each day, preparing and eating foods rich in antioxidants, and taking L-arginine and the other supplements that may very well transform your health. It is time to start following my recommendations and start caring for yourself.

I urge you to take this book with you to your next doctor's appointment, share some of what you have learned with your physician, and ask him if **Say Yes to NO** is for you. My guess is that he will cheer you on. Ask your doctor to look me up on my Web site: www.ignarro.com.

Once you are launched, be sure to keep him updated on how you feel and on your blood pressure readings, if you are monitoring them at home, which could reduce your need for prescription medications—as it has for so many people quoted in the book. In the process, lifestyle decisions you make today and in the weeks, months, and years ahead will dramatically affect your susceptibility to having a heart attack, a stroke, and many other serious cardiovascular conditions.

My wish for you—and the motivation for so much of my scientific research—is that you have a long, active, and enjoyable life. My objective is to help you maximize the activity of the nitric oxide in your body, which in turn will improve your cardiovascular well-being to a substantial extent.

IN PARTING

This chapter began with the sobering statistic that one out of two Americans will die of cardiovascular disease—which in most cases could have been prevented. You can beat those odds, even if you currently have high blood pressure, have suffered a heart attack, or are at high risk. The power to lead an entirely new and healthier life is in your hands. The sooner you get started, the sooner you will begin to see results in the way you feel and in your doctor's evaluation of your health status—very possibly in a matter of weeks.

There is a Latin maxim you have no doubt heard: *carpe diem*—seize the day. That is what I want you to do. Seize the day and start boosting your NO production right now. If you embark on the **Say Yes to NO** program, I would love to hear about the results you achieve. Let me know by sending an e-mail to SayYestoNO@NOMoreHeartDisease.com. I expect so many e-mails to come pouring in that my staff will not be able to reply to all of them.

RESOURCES

CHAPTER 1

Fant K. *Alfred Nobel: A Biography*. New York: Arcade, 1993.

Halasz N. *Nobel: A Biography of Alfred Nobel*. London: Orion, 1959.

Ignarro LJ (ed.). *Nitric Oxide: Biology and and Pathobiology*. San Diego: Academic Press, 2000.

Katsuki S, Arnold W, Mittal C, et al. Stimulation of guanylate cyclase by sodium nitroprusside, nitroglycerin and nitric oxide in various tissue preparations and comparison to the effects of sodium azide and hydroxylamine. *J Cyclic Nucleotide Res* 1977; 3:23–25.

Murad F, Mittal CK, Arnold WP, et al. Guanylate cyclase: activation by azide, nitro compounds, nitric oxide, and hydroxyl radical and inhibition by hemoglobin and myoglobin. *Adv Cyclic Nucleotide Res* 1978; 9:145–158.

CHAPTER 2

American Heart Association. *Heart Disease and Stroke Statistics—2003 Update,* 2003.

Houston MC. The role of vascular biology, nutrition and nutraceuticals in the prevention and treatment of hypertension. *JANA* 2000; Suppl 1:5–71.

Ongini E, Impagnatiello F, Bonazzi A, Guzzetta M, Govoni M, Monopoli A, Del Soldato P, and Ignarro LJ. Nitric oxide (NO)-releasing statin derivatives, a class of drugs showing enhanced antiproliferative and anti-inflammatory properties. *Proc Natl Acad Sci USA* 2004; 101:8497–8502.

CHAPTER 3

Ignarro LJ (ed.). *Nitric Oxide: Biology and Pathobiology.* San Diego: Academic Press, 2000.

CHAPTER 4

American Heart Association. *Heart Disease and Stroke Statistics—2003 Update,* 2003.

Houston MC. The role of vascular biology, nutrition and nutraceuticals in the prevention and treatment of hypertension. *JANA* 2000; Suppl 1:5–71.

Ignarro LJ (ed.). *Nitric Oxide: Biology and Pathobiology.* San Diego: Academic Press, 2000.

Ignarro LJ, Bush PA, Buga GM, et al. Nitric oxide and cyclic GMP formation upon electrical field stimulation cause relaxation of corpus cavernosum smooth muscle. *Biochem Biophys Res Commun* 1990; 170:843–850.

Sherman DL. Exercise and endothelial function. *Coron Artery Dis* 2000; 11:117–122.

CHAPTER 5

Aviram M. Review of human studies on oxidative damage and antioxidant protection related to cardiovascular diseases. *Free Radic Res* 2000; 33 (Suppl):S85–97.

Bode-Boger SM, Boger RII, Creutzig A, et al. *Clin Sci (Lond)* 1994; 87:303–310.

Boger RH, Bode-Boger SM, Thiele W, et al. Restoring vascular nitric oxide formation by L-arginine improves the symptoms of intermittent claudication in patients with peripheral arterial occlusive disease. *J Am Coll Cardiol* 1998; 32:1336–1344.

Diplock AT. Antioxidant nutrients and disease prevention: an overview. *Amer J Clin Nutrit* 1991; 53(1 Suppl):189S–193S.

Egashira K. Clinical importance of endothelial function in arteriosclerosis and ischemic heart disease. *Circ J* 2002; 66:529–533.

Hishikawa K, Nakaki T, Tsuda M, et al. Effect of systemic L-arginine administration on hemodynamics and nitric oxide release in man. *Jpn Heart J* 1992; 33:41–48.

Houston MC. The role of vascular biology, nutrition and nu-traceuticals in the prevention and treatment of hypertension. *JANA* 2000; Suppl 1:5–71.

Hurson M, Regan MC, Kirk SJ, et al. Metabolic effects of argi-nine in a healthy elderly population. *JPEN J Parenter Enteral Nutr* 1995; 19:227–230.

Kumar DV, Das UN. Are free radicals involved in the pathobiol-ogy of human essential hypertension? *Free Radic Res Commun* 1993; 19:59–66.

Lerman A, Burnett JC, Higano ST, et al. Long-term L-arginine supplementation improves small-vessel coronary endothelial function in humans. *Circulation* 1998; 97:2123–2128.

Maxwell AJ, Anderson BE, Cooke JP. Nutritional therapy for pe-ripheral arterial disease: a double-blind, placebo-controlled, ran-domized trial of HeartBar. *Vasc Med* 2000;5:11–19.

Romero-Alvira D, Roche E. High blood pressure, oxygen radi-cals and antioxidants: etiological relationships. *Med Hypotheses* 1996; 46:414–420.

Siani A, Pagano E, Iacone R, et al. Blood pressure and metabolic changes during dietary L-arginine supplementation in humans. *Am J Hypertens* 2000; 13(5 Pt 1): 547–551.

Wolf A, Zalpour C, Theilmeier G, et al. Dietary L-arginine supplementation normalizes platelet aggregation in hypercholesterolemic humans. *J Am Coll Cardiol* 1997; 29:479–485.

CHAPTER 6

Baggio E, Gandini R, Plancher AC, et al. Italian multicenter study on the safety and efficacy of coenzyme Q10 as adjunctive therapy in heart failure (interim analysis). The CoQ10 Drug Surveillance Investigators. *Clin Investig* 1993; 71(8 Suppl): S145–149.

Devaraj S, Li D, Jialal I. The effects of alpha tocopherol supplementation on monocyte function. Decreased lipid oxidation, interleukin 1 beta secretion, and monocyte adhesion to endothelium. *J Clin Invest* 1996; 98:756–763.

Enstrom JE, Kanim LE, Klein MA. Vitamin C intake and mortality among a sample of the United States population. *Epidemiology* 1992; 3:194–202.

Friedrich MJ. To "E" or not to "E," Vitamin E's role in health and disease is the question. *JAMA* 2004; 292:671–673.

Graham IM, Daly LE, Refsum HM, et al. Plasma homocysteine as a risk factor for vascular disease. The European Concerted Action Project. *JAMA* 1997; 277:1775–1781.

Kritchevsky SB, Shimakawa T, Tell GS, et al. Dietary antioxidants and carotid artery wall thickness. The ARIC Study. Atherosclerosis Risk in Communities Study. *Circulation* 1995; 92:2142–2150.

Langsjoen H, Langsjoen P, Langsjoen P, et al. Usefulness of coenzyme Q10 in clinical cardiology: a long-term study. *Mol Aspects Med* 1994; 15 Suppl:S165–175.

Panigrahi M, Sadguna Y, Shivakumar BR, et al. Alpha-lipoic acid protects against reperfusion injury following cerebral ischemia in rats. *Brain Res* 1996; 717:184–188.

Rimm EB, Stampfer MJ, Ascherio A, et al. Vitamin E consumption and the risk of coronary heart disease in men. *N Engl J Med* 1993; 328:1487–1489.

Schnyder G, Roffi M, Flammer Y, et al. Effect of homocysteine-lowering therapy with folic acid, Vitamin B_{12} and Vitamin B_6 on clinical outcome after percutaneous coronary intervention. *JAMA* 2002; 288:973–979.

Stampfer MJ, Hennekens CH, Manson JE, et al. Vitamin E consumption and the risk of coronary disease in women. *N Engl J Med* 1993; 328:1444–1449.

Stephens NG, Parsons A, Schofield PM, et al. Randomised controlled trial of Vitamin E in patients with coronary disease: Cambridge Heart Antioxidant Study (CHAOS). *Lancet* 1996; 347:781–786.

Vasdev S, Ford CA, Parai S, et al. Dietary alpha-lipoic acid supplementation lowers blood pressure in spontaneously hypertensive rats. *J Hypertens* 2000; 18:567–573.

CHAPTER 7

Anderson JW, Johnstone BM, Cook-Newell ME. Meta-analysis of the effects of soy protein intake on serum lipids. *N Engl J Med* 1995; 333:276–282.

Bierenbaum ML, Reichstein R, Watkins TR. Reducing atherogenic risk in hyperlipemic humans with flax seed supplementation: a preliminary report. *J Am Coll Nutr* 1993; 12:501–504.

Ferrara LA, Raimondi AS, d'Episcopo L, et al. Olive oil and reduced need for antihypertensive medications. *Arch Intern Med* 2000; 160:837–842.

Folts JD. Potential health benefits from the flavonoids in grape products on vascular disease. *Adv Exp Med Biol* 2002; 505:95–111.

Freedman JE, Parker C, Li L, et al. Select flavonoids and whole juice from purple grapes inhibit platelet function and enhance nitric oxide release. *Circulation* 2001; 103:2792.

Fuhrman B, Lavy A, Aviram M. Consumption of red wine with meals reduces the susceptibility of human plasma and low-density lipoprotein to lipid peroxidation. *Am J Clin Nutr* 1995; 61:549–554.

Haskell WL, Spiller GA, Jensen CD, et al. Role of water-soluble dietary fiber in the management of elevated plasma cholesterol in healthy subjects. *Am J Cardiol* 1992; 69:433–439.

Okuda Y, Kawashima K, Sawada T, et al. Eicosapentaenoic acid enhances nitric oxide production by cultured human endothelial cells. *Biochem Biophys Res Commun* 1997; 232:487–491.

Keenan JM, Pins JJ, Frazel C, et al. Oat ingestion reduces a systolic and diastolic blood pressure in patients with mild or borderline hypertension: a pilot trial. *J Fam Pract* 2002; 51:369.

Rein D, Paglieroni TG, Wun T, et al. Cocoa inhibits platelet activation and function. *Am J Clin Nutrit* 2001; 72:30–35.

Sirtori CR, Lovati MR. Soy proteins and cardiovascular disease. *Curr Atheroscler Rep* 2001; 3:47–53.

CHAPTER 8

Blair SN, Kohl HW, Paffenbarger RS, et al. Physical fitness and all-cause morality. A prospective study of healthy men and women. *JAMA* 1989;262:2395–2401.

Gielen S, Schuler G, Hambrecht R. Exercise training in coronary artery disease and coronary vasomotion. *Circulation* 2001; 103:E1–E6.

Hambrecht R, Fiehn E, Weigl C, et al. Regular physical exercise corrects endothelial dysfunction and improves exercise capacity in patients with chronic heart failure. *Circulation* 1998; 98:2709–2715.

Hardman AE, Hudston A. Brisk walking and serum lipid and lipoprotein variables in previously sedentary women—effect of

12 weeks of regular brisk walking followed by 12 weeks of detraining: *Br J Sports Med* 1994; 28:261–266.

Hornig B, Maier V, Dresler H. Physical training improves endothelial function in patients with chronic heart failure. *Circulation* 1996; 93:210–214.

Simon-Schnass I, Pabst H. Influence of Vitamin E on physical performance. *Int J Vitam Nutr Res* 1988; 58:49–54.

Taddei S, Galetta F, Virdis A, et al. Physical activity prevents age-related impairment in nitric oxide availability in elderly athletes. *Circulation* 2000; 101:2896–2901.

Tucker LA, Friedman GM. Walking and serum cholesterol in adults. *Am J Public Health* 1990; 80:1111–1113.

CHAPTER 9

Buga GM, Wei LH, Bauer PM, et al. NG-hydroxy-L-arginine and nitric oxide inhibit Caco-2 tumor cell proliferation by distinct mechanisms. *Am J Physiol* 1998; 275(4 Pt 2): R256–264.

Heinonen OP, Albanes D, Virtamo J, et al. Prostate cancer and supplementation with alpha-tocopherol and beta-carotene: incidence and mortality in a controlled trial. *J Nat Canc Inst* 1998; 90:440–446.

Johnstone MT, Creager SJ, Scales KM, et al. Impaired endothelium-dependent vasodilation in patients with insulin-dependent diabetes mellitus. *Circulation* 1993; 88:2510–2516.

Kruman II, Kumaravel TS, Lohani A, et al. Folic acid deficiency and homocysteine impair DNA repair in hippocampal neurons and sensitize them to amyloid toxicity in experimental models of Alzheimer's disease. *J Neurosci* 2002; 22:1752–1762.

Sano M, Ernesto C, Thomas RG, et al. A controlled trial of selegiline, alpha-tocopherol, or both as treatment for Alzheimer's disease. The Alzheimer's Disease Cooperative Study. *N Engl J Med* 1997; 336:1216–1222.

Yong LC, Brown CC, Schatzkin A, et al. Intake of Vitamins E, C, and A and risk of lung cancer. The NHANES I epidemiologic followup study. First National Health and Nutrition Examination Survey. *Am J Epidemiol* 1997; 146:231–243.

CHAPTER 10

Ignarro LJ (ed.). *Nitric Oxide: Biology and Pathobiology.* San Diego: Academic Press, 2000.

INDEX